Challenging Behaviour in DEMENTIA

Additional titles in the **Winslow Editions** series:

Counselling with Reality Therapy, Robert E Wubbolding & John Brickell

Person-Centred Approaches to Dementia Care, Ian Morton

Family Therapy with Older Adults & their Families, Alison Marriott

Beyond Aphasia: Therapies for Living with Communication Disabilities, Carole Pound, Susie Parr, Jayne Lindsay & Celia Woolf

Challenging Behaviour in DEMENTIA

A Person-Centred Approach

Graham
STOKES

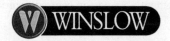

Winslow Press Ltd
Telford Road, Bicester, Oxon OX6 0TS, UK

First published in 2000 by
Winslow Press Ltd, Telford Road, Bicester, Oxon OX6 0TS, UK
www.winslow-press.co.uk

002-4207/Printed in the United Kingdom/1010

British Library Cataloguing in Publication Data
Stokes, Graham, 1952–
    Challenging behaviour in dementia : a person-centred approach. – (Winslow editions)
    1. Senile dementia
    I. Title
    616.8'983
ISBN 0 86388 250 1

*To Jayne, Liam, Rebecca and Georgina
who gave me treasured support during
the times I spent in my other place*

Graham Stokes is a Consultant Clinical Psychologist, Premier Health NHS Trust, Staffordshire, and Director of Mental Health, BUPA Care Services. He is a specialist in neurodegenerative disease and dementia, and has been instrumental in the development of person-centred approaches to assessment and care, with particular reference to challenging behaviour.

Among his publications are the series *Common Problems with the Elderly Confused* (Winlsow, 1986), *On Being Old: The Psychology of Later Life* (publisher, date) and (co-edited with Fiona Goudie) *Working with Dementia* (Winslow, 1990) a revised and updated version of which, *The Essential Dementia Care Handbook*, is due for publication by Winslow in 2001.

Contents

Figures

Tables

Preface

I NEVER INTENDED TO WORK IN THE FIELD OF DEMENTIA: to do so was to demonstrate either a lack of ambition or poor judgement; possibly, it was even evidence that you had done something wrong. It was an area of clinical activity that was disparaged and neglected. Are we talking of decades ago? No, this was the mid-1980s. For me the attraction was neuropsychology and the opportunity to research the psychological 'management' of dementia.

Within the space of just a few years, however, I found that my organic model was flawed and my interventions were not simply inadequate, but they appeared to betray the essence of dementia. At the core of our understanding was a need not to understand in ever greater detail the nature of brain disease, but to acknowledge the presence of a person. As a result of spending many hours in the company of those with dementia, it became evident that we do not 'work with dementia', but work with people whose intellectual powers are failing, yet who remain as you and I, sentient beings rich in need and feeling. Their actions and words had not been seen as the pathway to understanding, but were wrongly degraded to the status of symptoms, signs of an incurable disease. The outcome was interventions that resonated with a requirement to control and manage the ensuing problems. It is less than 20 years ago that the literature employed terms such as 'senile dements', or made reference to 'an undesirable symptom found in senility'.

The purpose of this book is to communicate the rapidly expanding knowledge of the psychology of dementia and how this has provided insights into the origins of challenging behaviour. Over the past decade our understanding has moved on to such an extent that it is now an exciting time to be working in the psychological care of people with dementia. Certainly there remain pockets of traditional practice dominated by a narrowly defined medical model, but overall the quality of dementia services has been transformed out of all recognition during the past 15 years. We are dismantling the asylums, rejecting the harshness of task-driven custodial care and abandoning the assertion that neuropathology explains all. In their place we find humanitarian concern and an empathic quest for answers. How well resourced is the person to cope with their dementia? What needs are being articulated in their speech and conduct? What role is the care setting playing in the genesis of their behaviour? There is an appreciation that quality care is the function of human relationships – no longer them and us, where we address their disability and, if not neglect, then relegate to a subordinate status their personhood. The person and their psychology remain, not to be ignored, but to be the guiding principle behind whatever we do to help them negotiate their harrowing journey into and through a world of not knowing. The person presents as very different, but it is misguided to use this as evidence for asserting that the person has departed, leaving behind an empty shell. Appearances may support such an assertion but, as they say, appearances can be deceptive.

This book starts with an understanding of the term 'dementia', identifying it as a clinical syndrome, not a disease. It establishes that the greatest burden of care is to be found, not in the realm of cognitive impairment, but in the domain of challenging behaviour; what the person has started to do, rather than what they can no longer do: wandering, noisemaking, abuse, violence, inappropriate toileting. These are, however, simply labels, and labelling bedevils mental healthcare in general, and dementia care in particular. Chapter 2 examines the issue of labelling and advocates a model of description that enables us to communicate precisely what a person is doing, rather than indulging in imprecise assessment.

Having acknowledged the nature of challenging behaviour, a person-centred model of understanding that addresses the subjective experience of dementia is developed over the next four chapters, a model that does not deny the contribution of neuropathology, but which also reveals a person, unique, yet with whom we have so much in common, an individual struggling to survive and communicate behind a barrier of intellectual and linguistic destruction. The model provides us with the raison d'être to reach out to the person behind the barrier and interpret their signals so we are able to recognise and meet their needs, rather than being party to their frustration.

The model of understanding implicates neurogenic, medical, psychological and environmental influences, and as such requires methodologies of enquiry. In Chapters 7 and 8 techniques are described that employ behavioural observation, inference and intuition to bring order to the information we unearth. Chapter 9 examines the potential of communication as a means of deciphering the words and behaviour of those with dementia, helping us to decode the cryptic messages. Resolution therapy is described and proposed as a means of achieving insights into the origins of demanding and disruptive behaviour. It does not represent a radical reinterpretation of human verbal communication, but acknowledges that the articulations of people with dementia are likely to mean something, and if we employ proven counselling qualities and skills that enable others to communicate more of themselves then we might learn something from their fragmented and seemingly incomprehensible speech.

The final chapters move us on from understanding to intervention: no longer 'management', but, in the first instance, resolution. Using case illustrations, an approach employed throughout the book, we see how challenging behaviour is resolved through the meeting of need. Toilet refusal, destructive behaviour, hoarding, nocturnal disturbance and aggression are some of the behaviours addressed through the introduction of person-centred care plans.

Psychological interventions to resolve challenging behaviour are in their ground-breaking infancy, and resolution is by no means always possible. A model of understanding is proposed that drives us towards the prospect of solution, but it is not a guarantee of success. Chapter 11 examines the skills necessary for working, not with 'symptoms' or 'problems', but with unmet need. Person-centred strategies to cope with abusive confrontations, violent assault and wandering are described and evaluated, as are methods not specific to any behaviour, namely distraction, behaviour modification, aromatherapy and the symptomatic use of medication.

Finally, the psychology of challenging behaviour concludes with the challenge of confusion. How do we bring peace of mind to those whose needs are experienced within the psychological reality of years past? Can we alleviate the torment of those who search for young children, seek their parents and want their home? The relative merits of reality orientation, time-shift, collusion and validation in modern dementia care are examined. The accepted practices of correction and deception are seen as less effective and potentially more distressing than interventions that address the subjective world of confusion and relate to the person and their feelings of anger, sadness and despair.

Today, it feels very different working in the field of dementia. Diagnosis nowadays incorporates both pathology and the person. As has been written elsewhere, a new culture of care is apparent. We endeavour to understand, we affirm the value of the person and their experience, and continually search for means of meeting need. The area attracts bright minds and innovation. The last decade or so has presented us with an illuminating and stimulating road along which to travel. I, for one, welcome the new millennium, a time when we may consolidate our clinical and care gains, achieve fresh insights, shatter more myths and enthuse those who remain to be convinced that words such as 'rehabilitation', 'potential', 'creativity' and 'resolution' truly belong to the language of dementia care.

Graham Stokes
June 2000

Acknowledgements

THIS BOOK IS DEDICATED TO the men and women with dementia, and the many family carers whom it has been my privilege to meet. We shared concerns, faced many struggles and negotiated occasional exasperation. Most of all, I valued the time they gave to share their experience and illuminate the meaning of their lives.

I wish to express my thanks to those colleagues who have informed and inspired my thinking, most especially Fiona Goudie, Gerald Hall, Una Holden and Mike Sherman. I also owe a great debt to the clinicians and professional caregivers with whom I have worked and taught over the years. Time and time again I unearthed a rich vein of knowledge born of unquestionable commitment. Please accept my thanks, even though I cannot list you by name.

Finally, I am grateful to Helen Hill and Sue Banting, who processed the manuscript with such unerring accuracy and were kind enough not to complain about my handwriting.

CHAPTER 1

Dementia: No Longer a 'Silent Epidemic'

O VER RECENT YEARS dementia in old age has acquired a depth of understanding among health and social care professionals that militates against the belief that confusion, intellectual decline and incompetence in the skills of daily living are inevitable accompaniments of ageing. While the prevailing cultural expectation still appears to be that mental infirmity is a normal feature of later life, the reality is that when marked cognitive impairment and behavioural change occurs in old age these are the result of disease. In other words, dementia is abnormal, not normal, and thus its origins are pathological and not the inevitable outcome of being old. Such knowledge, however, does not generate optimism among practitioners working with dementia. It remains a condition associated with inevitable and inexorable decline, disintegration and despair. Such pessimism is invariably indexed by therapeutic nihilism wherein hopes for rehabilitation and resolution of behaviour that is challenging are deemed to be objectives incompatible with the nature of the problem. The question this book addresses is whether this is necessarily so.

Dementia: Terminology

Although we speak of 'diagnosing' dementia (from the Latin 'demens', which means being out of one's mind) it is not a disease in its own right. It is an umbrella term employed to denote the existence of a neuropsychological syndrome: typically, memory impairment, intellectual deterioration, behavioural incompetence and social inadequacy. As such, dementia represents a clinical description without any supposition of an underlying aetiology (Wade & Hachinski, 1987).

Dementia: The Syndrome

For most of this century the appearance of dementia in old age did not warrant further investigations. The syndrome had been described as long ago as 1835, when James Cowles Prichard described 'senile dementia' as a state characterised by 'forgetfulness of recent impressions, while the memory retains a comparatively firm hold of ideas laid up in the recesses from times long past'. Similarly, Esquirol (1838) provided a clinical description which corresponds in many ways to current classification:

> Senile dementia is established slowly. It commences with enfeeblement of memory, particularly the memory of recent impressions. The sensations are feeble; the attention, at first fatiguing, at length becomes impossible; the will is uncertain and without impulsion; the movements are slow and impractical.

As intellectual deterioration and memory loss was considered to be an almost inevitable consequence of ageing, such developments were considered by many to be an extreme variant of normal age-related changes. If a neuropathological basis was required, the most common explanation was felt to be cerebral arteriosclerosis – 'hardening of the arteries'. The brain was seen to be starved of its blood supply, resulting in a progressive dementia. 'However, knowledge was disfigured by myth and distorted by disinterest' (Stokes, 1992).

Nowadays, however, the aetiology and classification of late-life dementia (the terms 'late-life' or 'late-onset' are favoured, not 'senile', for the latter is a pejorative description rich in stigma) are no longer neglected clinical issues. The Royal College of Physicians (1981) defined the syndrome as:

---

the global impairment of higher cortical functions including memory, the capacity to solve the problems of day-to-day living, the performance of learned perceptuomotor skills, the correct use of social skills and the control of emotional reactions in the absence of gross clouding of consciousness. The condition is often irreversible and progressive.

Cummings & Benson (1983) define dementia as an acquired and persistent impairment of intellectual function with deficits in at least three of the following spheres of mental activity: language, memory, visuospatial skills, emotion or personality, and cognition (abstraction; calculation, judgement, etc).

Jorm (1987) questions why we persist with the descriptive term of dementia which is non-specific as to causation, rather than focus on the specific conditions which give rise to it. These include Alzheimer's disease, dementia with Lewy bodies, multi-infarct dementia, Pick's disease, Creuzfeldt-Jakob disease and chronic alcohol abuse, which are themselves 'all referred to as dementia' (ibid). For example 'Dementia is a group of progressive diseases' (Murphy, 1986), 'dementia is a set of diseases of the brain' (Marshall, 1998) and 'Dementia is a disease' (Moniz-Cook, 1998).

The answer is that, when used judiciously, 'dementia' can be a useful concept. The presumptive causes of dementia are often hard to tell apart, especially in the early stages. A definite diagnosis is also impossible during life. It therefore can be seen as a 'compromise diagnosis', which acknowledges a set of characteristic signs and symptoms and excludes a range of alternative diagnoses. Figure 1.1 illustrates how the term 'dementia' is used as both a descriptor of intellectual and behavioural dysfunction, and an explanation for those decrements.

It is essential, however, to appreciate that the presence of cognitive deficits and behavioural incompetence cannot automatically be assumed to be evidence of dementia. The case of Mrs W illustrates the multifactoral nature of cognitive impairment in old age and how the term 'dementia' is often used injudiciously.

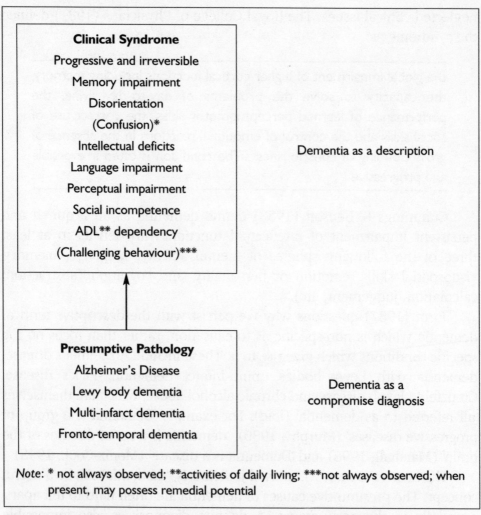

Figure 1.1 *Dementia: a descriptor of, and explanation for, dysfunctional cognition and behaviour*

Case Study: Mrs W
Client: Mrs W, aged 81 years
Diagnosis: Dementia of the Alzheimer type
Demographics: Widowed for 5 years. Lived alone
History:
I Over a two-year period noticed to be absent-minded, at times muddled and 'cantankerous'.

2 Admitted to a residential home six months ago as considered to be at risk.

3 Since entry to the home she has been observed to be subdued, withdrawn and increasingly disoriented.

4 Visited by a psychiatrist who asked such questions as day, date, town, county and the name of the prime minister and residential home. She was assessed using the Mini-Mental State Examination (MMSE). The MMSE has a series of tasks such as spelling a word backwards, recalling three objects or copying a design, that test a range of cognitive functions.

5 Poor performance, including a score of 11:30 on the MMSE, led to both an assumption of severe cognitive impairment and a diagnosis of dementia.

Reformulation

1 At the time of her interview and assessment Mrs W had been confined to bed for the previous six days with a chest infection.

2 Mrs W had been registered blind since 1981, and had worn a hearing aid since 1987.

Opinion
Ill-health and profound sensory disadvantage severely compromised her ability to comprehend her world, and significantly interfered with her capacity to respond to questions and perform tasks. A 'diagnosis' of dementia was both ill-founded and prejudicial.

The case of Mrs W illustrates that a reliable diagnosis of dementia can only follow accurate assessment of performance and the exclusion of physical morbidity, psychological disorder and sensory impairment that may also be responsible for cognitive decline and dependency in old age. Alternative explanations include delirium caused, for example, by chest infection, urinary tract infection, constipation and toxic states, including the effects of prescribed medication (see Pitt, 1987); treatable dementia resulting from brain tumour, vitamin B12 deficiency, hypothyroidism and subdural haematoma (Byrne, 1987); benign senescent forgetfulness (Kral, 1962; 1978) and severe depression (Jorm, 1987) – but not being old (Stokes, 1992). A 'diagnosis' of 'What do you expect at their age?' is both wrong and demeaning.

Dementia: Prevalence

Methodological Considerations

Recent prevalence studies estimate that there are 636,000 people in the United Kingdom with dementia (Alzheimer's Disease Society, 1995), yet, as there are no reliable ante-mortem markers for the most important causes of dementia, epidemiological studies rely on 'diagnoses' of dementia based upon clinical symptoms alone (Jagger & Lindesay, 1993). This immediately raises the question, 'What are the researchers measuring?' As we have seen, people may present with poor performance of cognitive function and incompetence in daily living for a variety of reasons. For example, the MMSE, mentioned above (Folstein *et al*, 1975) is a widely used screening instrument for the detection of cognitive impairment, yet Jagger & Lindesay (1993) note the number of studies that have demonstrated that a low level of education, extreme age, manual social class and visual impairments can cause subjects to be misclassified as cases of 'dementia'. Similarly, Henderson (1987) considers that the MMSE may not be applicable for those who 'have had little opportunity for education. Such brief screening measures do not allow a diagnosis of dementia to be made. Despite a general belief that they possess 'diagnostic value' (Pattie, 1988), these instruments are no more than measures of cognitive functioning and useful indicators of whether further investigations are necessary.

To address this methodological weakness, interest has been shown in a two-phase research design (Duncan-Jones & Henderson, 1978) wherein a relatively brief screening test (such as MMSE) is employed to screen out those people who are definitely *not* suffering from notable cognitive impairment. On the basis of their score on the screening test, the remainder are assessed more fully, usually by a clinician. Two of the second stage 'diagnostic' instruments in popular use are the Geriatric Mental State Examination (Copeland *et al*, 1976) and the Cambridge Mental Disorders of the Elderly Examination (Roth *et al*, 1988). It is to be expected that an epidemiological methodology that employs a two-stage approach to assessment will achieve appreciable gains in 'case identification' (that is, those people who have 'true' dementia). A review of the epidemiological methods and difficulties encountered in dementia research may be found in Jagger & Lindesay (1993).

Epidemiology
The great majority of dementia prevalence studies (of which there have been around 60 since 1945) have been conducted in Northern Europe, Japan and North America. Among the general population of people aged over 65, the prevalence rate (that is, the number of people with the disease at a given time divided by the number in the population at risk of acquiring the disease) of moderate and severe dementia (both points on a continuum of impairment rendering a person incapable of independent self-care) has generally been accepted to be between 5 and 8 per cent (Kay & Bergman, 1980).

Jagger & Lindesay (1993) consider that the norm in contemporary studies appears to be an overall rate in those aged 65 years and over of between 4 and 7 per cent. Detailed interpretation of epidemiological surveys is not justifiable, however, if for no other reason than that there are no standardised diagnostic criteria or interview instruments and so the information elicited about cases varies considerably between surveys (Henderson, 1987). There are no prevalence studies of dementia in Third World countries. As longevity is less common in developing countries, Henderson (1986) reports 'that dementia … is extremely rare'. As for those adults who enter old age, it is possible that they constitute a survival elite who may be resistant to the onset of dementia.

Mild dementia in old age has been estimated as having a prevalence rate between 1.5 and 21.9 per cent. As such great disparity makes clear, these figures for mild impairment of cognitive performance are unreliable and difficult to interpret. Kay & Bergmann (1980) conclude that mild dementia 'must be regarded as an experimental concept rather than a definite syndrome'.

Although prevalence estimates differ across studies, research always confirms the steep rise of dementia prevalence with age. It is estimated that around 17,000 younger people in the United Kingdom have 'early-onset dementia' (EOD), a term used to describe a syndrome which first begins before the arbitrary cut-off age of 65 years. Some sufferers will be only in their 20s or 30s (Alzheimer's Disease Society, 1995). Whalley *et al* (1982) suggested a prevalence rate of 0.1 per cent in people aged 45–64 years. In their study, Freyne *et al*, (1998) established a prevalence of 0.5 per cent in the 45–64 year age group, yet concluded 'this could well be an underestimate'. Jorm & Korten (1988) analysed data from 47 prevalence studies and estimated a rate of 0.7 per cent in the 60–64 year age group.

Findings of a collaborative reanalysis based on original data from European prevalence studies of dementia between 1980 and 1990 found a doubling of the prevalence with every five year age increase over 60 years up to 95 years of age (Hofman *et al*, 1991). This is in general agreement with estimates from studies conducted in other continents (for example Jorm *et al*, 1987). Table 1.1 illustrates the age distribution of dementia.

There are no major differences in prevalence of dementia between men and women, but as women are more likely to live into advanced old age (for example, 75 per cent of adults over 85 years are women) there are far more women with dementia than there are men.

As the prospect of developing dementia rises steeply in the eighth and ninth decades of life, the prevalence of dementia in society depends on the proportion of the population that survives to be very old. The marked increase in the number of people surviving into advanced old age

Table 1.1 *Pattern of dementia prevalence (%) by age*

Age (years)	Hofman et *al* (1991)	Jorm et *al* (1987)
60–64	1.0	0.7
65–69	1.4	1.4
70–74	4.1	2.8
75–79	5.7	5.6
80–84	13.0	10.5
85–89	21.6	20.8
90–94	32.2	38.6

(for example, in England and Wales in 1986 there were 639,000 people aged over 85 years; by 2006, the numbers will have reached 1,116,000) will produce what Henderson (1983) has called 'the coming epidemic of dementia'. Henderson & Jorm (1986), using population projections, anticipate that, over the period 1980 to 2000 there will have been an increase in the number of dementing people of 13 per cent in the United Kingdom, 41 per cent in the United States and 52 per cent in Australia. The epidemic of dementia will reach a peak when the babies of the boom years between 1945 and 1965 enter 'old age' from 2010 onwards. The World Health Organisation (1982) estimates that, between 1980 and 2020, the global growth in the over-65 population will be 150 per cent, rising from 260 million people to 650 million. The implications for the prevalence of dementia are profound.

Dementia: Incidence
Owing to problems of methodology and measurement there are very few studies of the incidence rate of dementia (the number of people developing a disease in a specified time period divided by the size of the population at risk). For example, Jorm (1990) reported only 12 incidence studies of dementia in old age.

Mortimer *et al* (1981) calculated an annual incidence rate of about 1 per cent in people aged 65 and over. Not surprisingly, the incidence of dementia rose sharply with age, from around 0.3 per cent at 65 years to approximately 3.5 per cent at age 85 years, in accordance with prevalence research. Mortimer (1983) suggests that there may be a decreased incidence of dementia in people aged over 90 years resulting from a selective survival effect.

As to the question whether dementia is nowadays more common, not because there are a greater number of older people, but because there is greater human vulnerability to the condition, there is little evidence from studies of incidence rates over time to suggest this is so. For instance, a study carried out in Sweden reported no significant difference in incidence rates between 1947 and 1957 and 1957 and 1972 (Rorsman *et al*, 1986).

It is unlikely that incidence studies will match the volume of studies conducted to measure the prevalence of dementia. The data are expensive and time consuming to obtain. With an approximate annual incidence rate of only 1 per cent, researchers would have to survey 1,000 people, involving both examination and re-examination, to identify just 10 new cases of dementia in a 12-month period!

Living with Dementia

Only the minority of elderly people with dementia live in hospital or other continuing care establishments. The vast majority of dementing people live in the community, supported by their family and friendship networks, some of whom are themselves elderly and infirm. As a consequence, studies examining the stress of caring have, in the main, concentrated on family caregivers. These informal carers make up the bulk of people who come into contact with people with dementia. Yet we should not forget that more than half of people aged over 80 live alone, most of them widows spending their last years of life unaccompanied by their spouse, and that around 30 per cent of elderly people never had children (Stokes, 1992). Who are the supporters of these people if they should dement?

The Cost of Caring

With the development of community care a significant objective of practitioners and their agencies has been 'to mobilize and maintain the effectiveness of informal support systems with the aim of maintaining a person with dementia at home' (Morris & Morris, 1993). However, this approach is not without cost for the informal carer. As Murphy (1991) writes, 'the "community" is not a real place, only a fictional ideal; the community is, in reality, overburdened families who have little choice'. Poulshock & Deimling (1984) have employed the term 'caregiving impact' to denote the effects of caring on health and family relationships, the primary expression of strain being in psychosocial impairment, rather than in physical or financial welfare. These effects are greater for carers caring for a relative with dementia than for those caring for a physically dependent relative (Eagles *et al,* 1987). Birkel (1987) found that caring for someone with dementia is generally much more difficult than assisting someone with physical care needs but few or no emotional or challenging difficulties.

Studies that have examined the effect of caring on psychological well-being report decreased morale and increased levels of depression and stress. Morris *et al* (1988) found that 15 per cent of their sample of spouse carers had levels of depression that were clinically significant. Pagel *et al* (1985) observed that 40 per cent of their sample were depressed. Pruchno & Resch (1989) identified stress and anxiety as further negative outcomes of caring, which may in turn be related to the increased incidence of health problems among caregivers. Feelings of anger may be a particularly important indicator of carer ill-being (Anthony-Bergstone *et al,* 1988). Both Bergmann & Jacoby (1983) and Gilleard *et al* (1984) found significant levels of probable 'caseness' of psychiatric disorder.

In contrast, Morris *et al* (1992) found low levels of depression in their sample of caregivers. Similarly, other studies have failed to demonstrate high levels of carer ill-being (for example, Eagles *et al*, 1987). While these studies may 'reflect the different levels of adaptation and impact of caring in people from different communities', Morris & Morris (1993) note that these disparate findings may be attributed to biases in the recruitment of carers to a study. For example, carers recruited through respite facilities may demonstrate more robust emotional health as 'something constructive is being done' to provide practical relief, while others may be subject to an unremitting and debilitating burden of care: what has been referred to as 'the 36-hour day' (Mace & Rabins, 1992).

In general, the severity of the cost of caring appears to be dependent on the closeness of the relationship between caregiver and the person with dementia. The less the familial distance, the greater the risk of depression and strain (for example, Gilhooly, 1984; George & Gwyther, 1986). Spouses are most likely to suffer problems of psychological health, followed by siblings and other family members. This is not difficult to appreciate, for the unremitting responsibility for care when combined with significant emotional involvement must be especially distressing (what a caring husband described as 'a tragic and distressing epilogue to our life of togetherness').

When depression is present it may arise from the uncontrollability of the caregiving demands. Morris *et al* (1989) found that, if carers experienced stress as unremitting with no prospect of solution, and this negative outlook permeated all aspects of their lives, this was predictive of depression. An alternative psychological variable mediating between caring and low mood may be the process of 'premature mourning' or 'anticipatory grief'.

The Objective and Subjective Burdens of Care

As behaviour changes during the course of dementia, the nature of the demands on caregivers also varies. This may be a further source of stress. Initially, carers may be faced with the devastation of higher level abilities that enable a person to carry out the roles of an independent adult (for example, taking responsibility for finances, household affairs, child care, transport and communication). Later, they will be confronted by the destruction of the basic activities of daily living, such as washing, toileting and dressing. There is also the prospect of having to cope with challenging behaviour, such as wandering, aggression and repetitive questioning, before having to provide continuous nursing care as the sufferer experiences the ultimate decline into an incoherent state of passive and total dependency.

Clearly, the *objective* burden of the carer varies in character during the months and years of caring. Yet do these experiences have equal potential to produce stress and strain? Do they all make life particularly difficult for the supporter? Can we equate the burden of having to constantly supervise someone who is at risk if they leave the house with the experience of no longer being able to hold a sensible conversation with them? Grad & Sainsbury (1965) adopted a distinction between *objective* and *subjective* burden. Objective burden is the practical impact of caregiving, such as performing intimate care tasks. Subjective burden is the emotional reaction to the objective burden of care. Some behavioural changes are less likely to be perceived as a problem, while others are experienced as problems that can precipitate, for instance, low morale, worry, anxiety, depression and despair. For example, while 29 per cent of supporters reported temper outbursts as a problem (Gilleard & Watt, 1982), Gilleard (1984) found a frequency of occurrence of almost 60 per cent: 'The objective recording of disabilities may be much less important, and is not the same as the subjective reporting of problems by supporters' (Gilleard, 1984).

The objective burden of caring is often elicited by 'symptom' checklists. Carers are then asked to rate the severity of these demands to determine their status as problems. Sandford (1975) found that nocturnal disturbance was a frequent complaint of family carers. Other problems included dangerous risky behaviour, incontinence and an inability to get in and out of bed. Greene *et al* (1982) examined the relationship between the degree of behaviour and mood disturbance, and the amount of stress and upset experienced by relative caregivers. These researchers concluded that carer distress was 'mainly a response' to the dementing person's passive withdrawn behaviour. Active disturbed behaviour was surprisingly found not to relate to carer stress. In a similar vein, Machin (1980) found carer strain to be related to a 'lack of behaviour', although she also observed over-demanding behaviour to be 'poorly tolerated'.

A series of research studies by Gilleard and his colleagues (for example, Gilleard & Watt, 1982; Gilleard *et al*, 1982) identified the frequency of behavioural deficits or excesses and their problem status for the carer. They found the greatest difficulties for supporters to be the need for constant supervision, night-time wandering, proneness to falls, incontinence and an inability to engage in meaningful activities. Unlike the challenging behaviours of incontinence and wandering, aggression was only cited as a 'great' problem by around a quarter of carers. Gilleard (1984) considers this may be because aggressive behaviours are 'occasional' rather than constant, and thus may be less significant sources of stress than, for example, the ever-present need for supervision. The problem status of aggressive behaviour is, however, equivocal. Other studies (for example, Lindesay & Murphy, 1989; Näsman *et al*, 1993) have linked carer strain and the failure of home support with 'aggression towards relatives'. Sheldon (1982) considered that wandering away from home causes the greatest anxiety. Agitated and repetitive behaviours in dementia are often rated as the most stressful for caregivers (Zarit & Edwards, 1996). In general, caregivers who have frequent behavioural or emotional problems to contend with are subject to greater stress (Pruchno & Resch, 1989). In contrast, cognitive impairment and the carer's having to assist a person with activities of daily living, including bathing, dressing and feeding, have generally been found not to be related to carer stress (Zarit & Edwards, 1996).

Overall, the common 'problems' that emerge from research on carer stress are incontinence, nocturnal disturbance, demandingness and apathy/withdrawal. 'Being restless and over-talkative during the day', 'wandering at night', 'calling out', 'being uncooperative and resistive', 'making accusations of ill treatment', 'causing trouble with the neighbours', 'interfering with others' possessions', 'engaging in destructive or embarrassing behaviour', 'hoarding', 'repeating the same request' or 'being followed from room to room' are easy to appreciate as the cause of intolerable strain. Withdrawal and an unwillingness to engage in conversation are possibly less easy to understand as potential sources of stress. Both types of behaviour are, however, evidence of a loss of rationality, comprehensibility and mutuality. The relationship ceases to be a relationship. There is no reciprocity and the person appears increasingly less like the person who was once known and loved. As a consequence, the behaviours serve 'to strain and endanger the bonds between dependant and caregiver' (Gilleard, 1984).

While it is tempting to analyse the strain of caring by reference to precise demands or an aggregate of discrete events, when talking to carers we find they often fail to describe specific problems, but instead talk about the unremitting toil of their daily existence. As a consequence, Lazarus & Delongis (1983) focus on what they term 'daily hassles'. These are described as the 'irritating, frustrating, distressing demands and troubled relationships that plague people day in and day out ... Some of which are transient, others repeated as even chronic.' Seeing the life of a carer as constituting 'daily hassles' may be more profitable than a perception of the caring role as comprising distinct stressful life events. In other words, the strain of caring is often greater than the sum response to specific instances of challenging behaviour. Often demands accumulate and merge one into the other, so that carers have little time to reflect on what is happening. They are confronted simply with the 'daily hassles' of being a carer.

The development of a one-sided unrewarding relationship can be seen as the distinguishing feature between caring for a person with dementia and caring for somebody with a physical illness. Caring for a relative with physical disabilities is demanding, but it can generate a reciprocal bond cemented by understanding, consideration and mutual respect. The behavioural problems in dementia are invariably experienced as unpredictable and baffling and project a lack of concern on the part of the dementing person. A loss of the relationship and a feeling of being trapped by one's responsibilities 'role captivity', may lead to the carer becoming physically or emotionally depleted by their caregiving obligations.

Summary

Several studies have reported that the major predictors of the breakdown of home support for dementing people 'are the levels of stress and well-being felt by principal caregivers' (Jerrom *et al*, 1993). While some studies have failed to establish an association between challenging behaviour and high levels of stress and psychiatric morbidity among carers (for example, Zarit *et al*, 1986), there is a strong body of evidence that has reported a positive relationship (for example, Gilleard *et al*, 1984; Kinney & Paris Stephens, 1989). Not surprisingly, families are more likely to seek help because of crises created by behavioural disturbances than by intellectual impairment in itself (Barnes & Raskind, 1980; Chenoweth & Spencer, 1986; Silver & Yudofsky, 1987).

The purpose of this book is to understand and resolve a principal source of carer strain, psychiatric referral, hospitalisation and demand for secure living arrangements, namely those challenging behaviours that dissolve a caregiver's capacity to cope: behaviours such as wandering, inappropriate toileting, aggression and passive retreat.

As the population ages, dementia is a growing social and healthcare problem. The financial challenge is huge (estimated in the United Kingdom to be around £6.1 billion each year), but in terms of emotional strain and physical exhaustion so is the price paid by caring families.

CHAPTER 2

Assessment of Behaviour in Dementia

DEMENTIA IS CHARACTERISED by changes in behaviour and cognition that are notoriously difficult to define. We have seen that challenging behaviour often presents carers with the greatest subjective burden. It is the most common reason for specialist intervention, treatment with psychotropic medication and hospitalisation (Steele *et al*, 1990). But what is meant by challenging behaviour? What is being communicated when we say, for example, a person with dementia 'wanders', or is said to be 'aggressive' or 'confused'? These are legitimate questions, for these terms are nothing more than subjective and imprecise labels. Despite operating under the guise of clinical credibility and quasi-scientific respectability, they are not incontrovertible behavioural phenomena. They are simply vague descriptions of action, rarely able to provide accurate and meaningful descriptions of behaviour. As such, they invariably lead to misunderstanding and self-fulfilling expectations (see Inness, 1998).

Behavioural assessment is dedicated to the accurate description of performance deficits and excesses, yet whether interview-based rating scales (for example, Hope & Fairburn, 1992), behaviour rating scales (for example, Pattie & Gilleard, 1979) or direct observation (for example, Bowie & Mountain, 1993) – the gold standard of behavioural assessment (Barlow & Hersen, 1984) – have been employed, most studies of challenging behaviour have been seriously handicapped by the practice of ill-defined labelling that masquerades as meaningful description. For example, weight loss is frequently observed in dementia (Seth, 1994) and is included in the clinical criteria for diagnosing Alzheimer's disease (McKhann et al, 1984). This may be a consequence of an eating problem, yet how often is this behaviour observed? Source material yields prevalence rates of 26 per cent (Morris et al, 1989), 13 per cent (Trinkle et al, 1992), 46 per cent (Swearer et al, 1988) and 10 per cent (Burns et al, 1990c). These marked disparities are, however, likely to reflect differences in the way in which the terms 'oral behaviour', 'abnormal eating behaviour', 'dietary change' and 'binge eating' were employed. Agitation is observed in dementia, yet Cohen-Mansfield et al, (1989) showed that the term covered excessive walking, aspects of aggressive behaviour, shouting, repeated plucking and 'any other behaviour which does not conform to norms of social conduct'.

Similarly, Haddad & Benbow (1993b) emphasise the need to avoid inappropriately labelling a person as having a 'sexual problem' on the basis of conduct that may in fact be non-sexual. For example, a person with dementia who climbs into bed with someone else, removes their clothes, exposes themselves in a communal lounge or walks around with their clothing inappropriately arranged may be erroneously labelled as having a 'sexual problem' when their conduct may have more to do with disorientation, discomfort, a toileting difficulty or a dressing apraxia (see Holden, 1990a; 1995).

Sexual misconduct has been described by Jensen (1989) as inappropriate sexual speech, hugging, kissing, self-exposure and attempted fondling. Haddad & Benbow (1993a) also include erotomania, morbid jealousy, public masturbation and excessive sexual demands. Furthermore, they acknowledge that 'a person with dementia may be incapable of going through the usual social and physical stages of sexual behaviour with their partner.' As a result, sexual intercourse may be clumsily attempted and actions taken to prevent participation in sexual relationships. It may even be the case that viewing sexual behaviour as unwanted might reflect the misconception that old age is a time of greatly diminished sexual interest and capacity (see Stokes, 1992). As a result, any sexual behaviour in dementia may be interpreted as deviant and thus experienced as a problem.

Despite the anticipatory concerns of both family and professional caregivers, and the range of behaviours embraced by the term 'sexual problem', it is a relatively uncommon challenging behaviour. Sourander & Sjogren (1970) did not define their use of the term, and reported a rate of 17 per cent, while Burns *et al*, (1990c) saw 'sexual disinhibition' (defined as obscene sexual language, masturbation, exposure and propositioning others) in 7 per cent of their sample.

Before we are able to understand challenging behaviour and intervene to resolve that behaviour, we must first define the nature of the 'problem'. We must employ a descriptive language that is meaningful and unambiguous. Two or more people must be able to know what a person has done following the communication of the description. Labels rarely, if ever, achieve this objective. They are economical to employ, but fail to define accurately the nature of the behaviour we wish to describe.

What is Behaviour?

'Behaviour' refers to observable acts which can be recorded and measured. This is known as a topographical definition of behaviour (Barlow & Hersen, 1984) and covers not only what a person does, but what they also say. With concepts such as memory impairment, failure of reasoning or loss of judgement, we infer such deficits from what somebody does or does not do. So a person is known to be forgetful when they mislay household items or fail to do what was intended. Yet what to count, for example, as forgetful or confused behaviour is by no means straightforward. As with observable actions such as 'aggression' and 'wandering' we continue to inhabit a world of labels. Despite their use as clinical signs, there is considerable disagreement as to what range of behaviour is to be included.

The American Psychiatric Association (1980) requires the presence of memory impairment when diagnosing dementia, without further specification being provided, yet there is 'a no-man's land where it is unclear at what point normal ends and abnormalities begin' (U'Ren, 1987). As Huppert & Tym (1986) observe, the large range of competence within the population of elderly people makes the 'determination of a threshold level of morbidity very difficult'. In truth, the characteristic signs of dementia are invariable dimensional, not categorical. The result may be that the cut-off point between what is considered 'normal', and thus acceptable and abnormal is arbitrary. And, as we will see, this may say more about the inadequacies of the person who is the assessor than about the individual who is being assessed.

Similarly, Byrne (1987) notes that an established criterion for the 'diagnosis' of dementia is intellectual impairment, yet 'this is not defined or quantified and so immediately raises the questions: what is intellectual impairment and at what level does it become pathological?'

Labels may be economical to employ, but are no more than imprecise judgements that resonate subjective interpretation. We may employ the same words, but it cannot be said that we always share a common language. Unfortunately, for some a diagnosis of dementia may represent little more than layering one ill-defined label upon another.

A Tripartite Model of Assessment

To address the inadequacy of much that passes for behavioural description, I advocate a tripartite model of assessment that starts with 'the label' then progresses to the formulation of an operational definition (Stokes, 1995a). While it is advisable to refrain from unthinkingly labelling a person's behaviour, because of the economy of effort involved it is unrealistic to hope that the practice of labelling will cease (although it should go without saying that those which are pejorative should be abandoned: for example, *senile* dementia). As labels can never offer a precise and unambiguous description of behaviour they should, however, be used with caution and be regarded as the first step towards a meaningful assessment.

The operational definition is rich in accurate descriptive detail and is composed of two elements. The behavioural definition is a precise description of the essential details and parameters of the troublesome behaviour. It avoids 'fuzzy', imprecise statements that are open to subjective interpretation. It is succinct and unambiguous, revealing the observable nature of the 'problem'. The process of defining a behaviour may involve a staff group 'brainstorming' what is meant by a particular label (for example, 'wandering', 'aggressive', 'confused') and then drawing up a behavioural definition that is based on the agreed description of the behaviour. The label can then be used with confidence, as everybody involved in the person's care knows what is meant by the term, and its use will be challenged if it is employed otherwise. It is thus being used in a considered fashion, rather than unthinkingly.

The behavioural characteristics constitute a description of 'what the behaviour looks like'; in other words, what the person actually does. In the practice of assessment and care, a client's behaviour would be described in terms unique to them and their circumstances: a process known as *pinpointing*. However, at a general level of description we can employ categories that are broad, but self-explanatory, manifestations of the challenging behaviour. Both the behavioural definition and characteristics constitute the operational definition – a definition that precisely details the behaviour in question and enables us to move on from understanding the nature of the action to an appreciation of the explanation. As we achieve an ever more fine-grained description of the person's behaviour we may, but will not always, embark upon a transition from 'what are they doing?' to 'why is it happening?' And when we move beyond the cognitive paradigm the explanations are rich and varied, and may have little to do with dementia.

We will now explore how this tripartite model of behavioural assessment builds upon some of the most commonly employed labels in dementia.

Forgetful: Aren't we All?

What do we Remember, What do we Forget?
As has already been noted, memory impairment is at the core of what is known as dementia. Yet to forget is part of the human condition. So are memory failures experienced in daily life, such as mislaying possessions, forgetting somebody's name, not remembering what you intended to do next (known as prospective memory loss), signs of incipient pathology or simply the product of a fallible memory?

How does Memory Work – Is there a Problem at All?
Considering less experimental studies that measure memory performance in the laboratory, but instead addressing memory function in everyday life, we need to bear in mind three essential principles. First, the natural state of affairs is not to remember: not to forget, but not even to

remember. We are bombarded with information throughout our working day, yet we retain only a fraction of what we experience. What happens to the rest? We do not forget it, we do not even bother to expend psychological energy remembering it. Within moments of the end of a favourite television programme, how much do you remember? Very little. Yet you followed the storyline, heard every word, and watched every scene. When you watch the news, is it all there at the end – every item, all the detail? By no stretch of the imagination is this so. Consider your day so far: how much can you remember? Of course, there is a sketch outline, but in what depth? Where is the richness of sequence and detail? How much of this book are you remembering?

It is not the case that we forget this variety of experience, instead we deem much of everyday life as not worthy of remembering. It is of no lasting significance or relevance, and thus we do not need to retain it. It is sufficient to perceive it, hold the information in temporary storage (known as working memory) so we are able to understand, appreciate and possibly respond to the experience, and then it fades away, never to be retrieved, for the moment was never retained.

The second principle is that we choose to remember and when we do, we expend energy and effort storing that information. What we choose to remember is whatever we consider to be necessary, significant or relevant to our lives. It may be practical or emotional. We all need to know where we have placed items and what bills to pay, but it is also pleasant to recall good times or have the knowledge never to repeat an unpleasant experience again. While there is much that we hold in common when considering what we need to remember, there is also much that is unique and idiosyncratic: information that has little relationship with the essentials of life, but instead reflects interests and passions.

The process of retaining information is known as 'encoding'. Experience is stored as a representation that relates to existing knowledge frameworks, while retaining distinctive contextual characteristics that identify its origin. In other words, a rich tapestry of association and detail is created. If the tapestry is threadbare, the associations weak, recall is difficult. Just because we decide that an experience is of value and hence needs to be remembered, it is no guarantee that the information will be recalled when it is next required. In other words, everybody's memory is fallible. This is forgetfulness. We do not condemn or label ourselves as forgetful if what we cannot recall was of no consequence. Such information has not been forgotten, it was not in the first place remembered. Only when we cannot recall an experience that was of personal or practical significance are we forgetful, for we know that it should have been stored for later retrieval. As an illustration of this distinction, where are your car keys? Where is your wallet, purse or bag? If at this point concern is surfacing, you are appreciating the significance of the information you cannot retrieve. Failure to recall will provide evidence of forgetfulness. Now ask yourself how many mouthfuls of food you consumed during your evening meal? Do not know? Forgetful? Of course not, the information was not worth remembering.

Finally, we come to the third principle of everyday memory. The meaningfulness and hence relevance, of experience ebbs and flows as we travel on life's journey. As we progress through life, as we shed and acquire responsibilities, adopt new lifestyles and roles, move in and out of relationships, the significance of information is not constant. For example, our daily lives are indexed by change, so we need to know the day and time, but how relevant is this information to a 79-year-old woman who has been a patient on an orthopaedic ward for seven weeks, housebound for two years, or who has lived in a residential home for 18 months? I suggest it is of little value. And what do we do with information that is of little consequence? Reject it as not worthy of remembering. Have you ever lost track of the days while on holiday? Did you terminate your vacation and head back to see your family doctor? Surely not. So why do we persist in determining an older adult's degree of memory impairment and disorientation by asking such questions as what is the day, month and year? How meaningful is this information to the daily lives of many older people? Why do we ask them who is the British prime minister or the president of the United States, the name of the British monarch or the heir to the throne? Why should such information be at the forefront of an older adult's mind? Are these burning issues to be addressed in everyday life? Ask yourself, who is the secretary general of the United Nations? How many nations are there in the European Union? Who is the prime minister of Canada? All feature in news broadcasts on television and radio, and appear in newspapers. But if you do not know the answers, have we evidence of forgetfulness? Or will you say, 'I am not interested, the information is irrelevant, and so not worth remembering'?

While we might like older adults to remain informed and have contact with the wider world, we must appreciate how meaningless much of it is to their daily existence. When we also appreciate that life becomes more effortful as we age and lose speed, strength and stamina (see Stokes, 1992) then it is to be expected that elderly people may conserve energy by encoding and thus remembering only that which is essential to life. So what do we learn when an older adult is unable to tell us the time, the day or the name of the prime minister, other than that we may have indulged in asking irrelevant questions that are likely to lead us to erroneous conclusions. So what are we to make of the guidelines for the use of the Information/Orientation subtest of the Clifton Assessment Procedures for the Elderly (Pattie & Gilleard, 1979; see Box 2.1)? A cut-off score of seven or below was originally suggested to indicate 'dementia', but later work suggested that eight or below detects moderate and severe 'dementia' (Brayne & Calloway, 1989; Clarke *et al*, 1991). Yet how many of these questions are meaningful and relevant to the daily experience of old age? Can they determine 'forgetfulness', and then be used as criteria for the diagnosis of dementia?

Box 2.1 Information/Orientation subtest of the Clifton Assessment Procedures for the Elderly (Pattie & Gilleard, 1979)

Name	Address	Colour of British flag
Age	City	Day
Date of birth	Prime minister	Month
Place	US president	Year

Even when asking autobiographical questions, such as 'date of birth', failure 'to know' may reflect not so much 'forgetfulness' as the loss of a memory trace through non-usage. How much do you remember of your school years? What is Pythagoras' theorem? πr^2? Co_2? The capital of Australia? The date Columbus 'discovered' America? Or the names of Henry VIII's six, or was it seven, wives? Are you now acknowledging the depth of your memory impairment, facing up to a 10-year partial amnesia, or are you simply saying, 'What do I need to know that for?' Life moves on, needs change, and through non-usage the memory trace withers on the vine. Maybe a day comes when your date of birth, the names of your siblings or when you left school acquire similar status. This appreciation of memory and the passage of time clearly undermines the significance of the question, 'How old are you? If the relevance of the year is questionable, and your date of birth may also become so, how are you able to calculate your age? The question itself falls into disrepute. Rather than focusing on eliciting somebody's precise age, the enquiry may be better conceived if it addresses the stage of life a person has reached. If a 78-year-old man reports that he is 69-years-old, this is acceptable. He does not know his age, but he knows his stage of life. His beliefs and actions will be appropriate. It would be different if he said he was 29. He might then have a young wife, small children, parents who are alive and a job to go to. His understanding and conduct would be discordant with current reality. This will not occur if he knows himself 'to be old'.

In summary, if you are party to an assessment that is subjecting an elderly person to the standard questions of information and orientation, respectfully enquire of the assessor if they know the names of the seven dwarves in the story of Snow White. If they express incredulity and fail to see the relevance of the question to the task at hand, I believe you may have successfully captured the inadequacy of the assessment.

The Operational Definition

Where does this leave us? It has taken us to an appreciation that a definition of forgetfulness, and thus a test of memory impairment, must address information that is of significance. Just because a person does not know the name of the prime minister, or even what day it is, it does not automatically follow that they cannot function independently. Carrying out domestic chores, taking medicine or knowing the telephone number of a caring daughter are not dependent on knowing the identity of the current incumbent of the White House. If the information or experience has value and significance, it may well be retained, even though awareness of many aspects of life is absent. And it is to the ability to survive in daily life that we now turn in order to provide the term 'forgetfulness' with its defining characteristic.

Operational Definition

Behavioural Definition
Forgetfulness is an inability to remember, as evidenced by action or speech, information necessary for the safe and satisfactory performance of the essential activities of daily life.

Behavioural Characteristics
The characteristics of forgetfulness are as follows:

- unable to recall essential telephone numbers or where they have been written down,
- mislaying household items,
- unable to remember messages,
- unable to remember appointments,
- cannot remember plans and intentions,
- cannot follow the thread of a conversation,
- repetitious speech content,
- does not remember to turn off taps or appliances (for example, cooker, gas fire),
- does not know the identity of significant others,
- unable to remember whether visitors have been,
- cannot locate the toilet or bedroom in their home,
- lost within a 'known' building,
- unable to recall present living arrangements,
- cannot recall whether they have eaten or medication has been taken,
- cannot remember to dress appropriately to context,
- unable to recall the purpose of action (the goal).

Having defined the characteristics of forgetfulness, if conversation or observation reveals the required evidence, we can proceed to the question of the cause: dementia or alternative pathology. Before we do so, however, a word of caution is in order. Even when information is objectively considered to be of significance, it can only be retained and recalled if the knowledge has been first conveyed. If an older adult lives an isolated life, or lives in institutionalised surroundings, the pertinent question is not so much, does the older adult 'know', as are they under-stimulated and disempowered, to an extent that such information is rarely, if ever, communicated?

Toileting Difficulty: Not Incontinence

Is incontinence an early-onset problem in dementia? In most cases the answer is 'no'. Are toileting difficulties to be expected early in the process of decline? For many people the answer is 'yes'. Are these incompatible responses to the same question, or is there a distinction between a toileting difficulty and incontinence?

One of the most difficult and distressing behaviours carers have to face is when a person with dementia starts to urinate in the 'wrong' places (Gilleard, 1984). It causes embarrassment and anger, and results in a heavy burden of physical care responsibility. Yet why is it that such problems arise relatively early in some people, when for others it presents towards the end of a slow process of cognitive and behavioural decline? As we shall see in Chapter 7, there is no simple answer to this question, for the achievement and maintenance of continence is a complex skill. However, what can be said with confidence is that when a person is found to be 'wet' or 'soiled', it is ill advised to label them automatically as incontinent. Incontinence denotes a failure of the controls associated with the normal storage of urine and results in the involuntary passing of urine. It is therefore an explanation for impaired toileting, not a description of that behaviour.

A failure to toilet may also arise even when bladder function is unimpaired. Stokes (1987a) referred to this as inappropriate urinating. This is characterised by an awareness of a need to urinate that does not result in the acceptable passing of urine. In other words, a person may still wet their clothes and furnishings despite possessing bladder control. It is thus premature to label an inability to toilet successfully as incontinence *unless* it is known that lost or damaged bladder control is the *explanation*.

If we must label the behaviour of a person who wets themselves, the term 'toileting difficulty' is preferable, for its usage logically leads on to the next question: 'why'? But, before we examine possible explanations, it has to be acknowledged that describing a person's behaviour as constituting a 'toileting difficulty' has, as yet, not offered us a precise and unambiguous description of behaviour. It remains an economical term open to misunderstanding and exploitation for, as a label, it cannot accurately define the nature of the dependency.

Box 2.2 shows how the tripartite model of assessment is applied to the impairment of toileting skills.

Box 2.2 The tripartite model of assessment

	OPERATIONAL	
Label	O	Toileting difficulty
	P	
Behavioural definition:	E R A T I O N	The voiding of urine or faeces either following an unsuccessful effort or with no apparent attempt to employ an acceptable facility (eg, toilet, commode, urine bottle)
Behavioural characteristics:	A L	Parcelling (eg, wrapping and concealing the evidence in drawers, cupboards, etc)
	D E	Wetting or soiling clothes while sitting (passive)
	F I	Wetting or soiling clothes while standing (active)
	N	Wetting or soiling the bed (passive)
	I	Using an inappropriate receptacle
	T	(eg, waste bin, fire bucket, plant pot)
	I	Urinating against wall
	O	Smearing
	N	

The behavioural definition does not discriminate on the basis of presumed intent, but focuses on the deficient toileting actions. The behavioural characteristics reveal how the defined behaviour was acted out, for example passive or active, discreet or invasive. 'Smearing' or 'parcelling' would be examples of invasive conduct. These descriptions, as with all attempts to establish taxonomies of descriptive characteristics, are the bare bones of the methodology. Each practitioner will need to clothe the skeleton differently according to the individual toileting characteristics of the person with dementia.

Aggressive: Violent, Offensive or Assertive?

Aggression is one of the most serious challenging behaviours associated with dementia (for example, Petrie *et al*, 1982; Colerick & George, 1986; Ryden, 1988; Näsman *et al*, 1993). Patients with dementia account for a significant majority of assaults and aggressive conduct in elderly in-patient settings (Patel & Hope, 1992a). The question of what to label as aggressive behaviour is, however, by no means straightforward.

In a study that associated violence with dementia, Shah (1992) defined violence 'as any act of physical aggression involving physical contact'. The levels of violence observed were low and the severity of injury from assaults mild. Clearly, the high prevalence of aggression in dementia is the consequence of behaviour other than physical assault. Ware *et al*, (1990) reported that aggressive behaviour caused great distress to carers despite the absence of physical violence. Several researchers (for example, Lion *et al*, 1981; Shah, 1991) believe that the under-reporting of aggressive behaviour is in part the result of the term being so ill-defined, and hence covering a range of quite distinct behaviours, that observer perception and tolerance of threat dominate reporting behaviour (see Inness, 1998). A study by Dean *et al* (1993) noted that an increase in 'aggressivity' reported by staff was accounted for by residents being 'better able to express themselves and make demands'.

Accepting that the most difficult boundary concerns verbal aggression, Patel & Hope (1993) suggest the following definition of aggressive behaviour: 'Aggressive behaviour is an overt act, involving the delivery of noxious stimuli to (but not necessarily aimed at) another object, organism or self, which is clearly not accidental.' The noxious stimulus can be either verbal or physical, but a question must be raised as to whether threat (for example, raising a fist, or spoken intent) is easily accommodated within the definition.

Factor analysis supports a distinction between verbal abuse, physical aggression and 'antisocial behaviour' (Patel & Hope, 1992a). Being uncooperative or resisting help (for example, pushing people away when they offer assistance), irritability and verbal abuse are the most common types of aggressive behaviour (ibid). When physical aggression is observed it manifests itself most commonly as biting, scratching, kicking and hitting (Hope & Patel, 1993), which on occasions can be dangerous (Ware *et al*, 1990). Destructive acts and sexual aggression are rare. Patel & Hope (1993) review observer rating scales that have been specifically designed to measure aggressive behaviour, including the Rating Scale for Aggressive Behaviour in the Elderly (RAGE) (Patel & Hope, 1992b).

Operational Definition

Behavioural Definition
Aggressive behaviour is injurious conduct involving the delivery of verbal abuse, or the threat or actual act of physical assault, spite or destruction to property, which is unquestionably non-accidental.

Behavioural Characteristics
Such characteristics may include the following:

spitting	tripping	damage to property
hitting	pinching	destroying property
biting	pushing	
slapping	nudging	
scratching	jabbing with elbow	swearing
kicking		insults
using an object to hit another	threatening to harm	being sarcastic and derogatory
physical resistance to care		yelling at another blaming and accusing

The characteristics incorporated within the definition *exclude* the following:

- irritability: an emotional state that is ill-defined and questionably observed;

- being uncooperative – may represent an unwillingness that is a legitimate act of assertiveness and thus to be respected;
- self-harm – an act worthy of consideration in its own right.

An accurate and agreed definition of aggressive behaviour is essential for appropriate understanding and intervention. If the assessment is inadequate the potential outcomes are misguided labelling, ill-advised interventions and the inappropriate use of psychotropic medication.

Wandering: We Walk, They Wander!

Most reports of the prevalence of wandering in dementia are flawed by the lack of both a clear definition of the behaviour and a reliable method of assessment. It is possibly the most misused and abused descriptive label employed in the area of challenging behaviour.

'Wandering is often one of the first symptoms that gets an individual living in the community into trouble, or puts him or her in danger' (Burnside, 1980). Rabins *et al*, (1982) reported that 40 per cent of family carers found wandering to be a troublesome problem. For those carers who find the need to provide constant supervision stressful, the strain can promote a range of coping strategies as extreme as physical restraints, chemical control (medication and alcohol) and 'aggression' (Dodds, 1994). Yet what is meant by wandering?

Hope & Fairburn (1990) believe that the term is used to cover such a wide range of walking behaviour that any attempt to define wandering will be unsuccessful. Instead, they propose a descriptive typology of wandering derived from interview data with carers. The classification incorporates a range of walking behaviour (for example, trailing a carer, aimless walking, walking for an inappropriate purpose) indexed by frequency, time and outcome (for example, needs to be brought back home). Hope *et al*, (1994) suggest the term 'abnormal walking around' to express the interrelatedness of certain types of wandering behaviour (namely, checking/trailing; excessive activity/aimless walking; pottering; inappropriate/over-appropriate [appropriate goal, excessive frequency] walking).

Contrary to the argument that wandering defies definition, Fisher & Carstensen (1990) define wandering as 'restless or aimless ambulation that is undesirable, because it results in the individual becoming lost, leaving an area of safety, getting into others' belongings, or because it interferes with more adaptive behaviours (eg, eating)'. This definition focuses on agitated and purposeless movement, and does little to address 'pottering' and other purposeful walking behaviour.

Operational Definition

Behavioural Definition
Wandering is a single-minded determination to walk that is unresponsive to persuasion: (a) with no or only superficial awareness for personal safety (for example, an inability to return; impaired recognition of hazard); or (b) with no apparent regard for others (for example, in terms of time of day, duration, frequency or privacy); or (c) with no regard for personal welfare (thereby disrupting the essential behaviours of eating, sleeping, resting).

The behavioural definition distinguishes between wandering with risk (a) and wandering as nuisance (b) as well as interpreting walking as wandering if the behaviour is 'to excess' (c), even though there is no risk or disturbance to others. The final element of the definition accommodates the finding that, following entry to a secure environment to live alongside others who rarely, if ever, respond, a person's 'abnormal walking' is relegated to the status of an unacknowledged behaviour, for their actions are less likely to trigger the threshold of concern. The absence of risk or nuisance should not, however, generate complacency or inertia to the point where the pursuit of understanding and resolution is deemed unnecessary.

Without this definition, the behavioural characteristics listed below (some of which are common to those established in the community survey of Hope & Fairburn, 1990) may attract the label of 'wandering' as soon as a person with dementia walks. The restrictions on activity that may follow can in turn result in a sedentary lifestyle and actions that may even contravene basic human rights (Mayer & Darby, 1991). Without doubt, the equation to avoid is that if wandering equals walking, then walking must equal wandering (see Box 2.3).

Box 2.3

An inadequate concept of wandering may lead to unnecessary and inhumane restrictions on activity.

Wandering equals walking, so

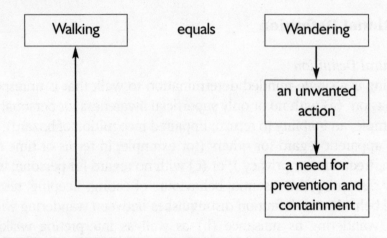

Behavioural Characteristics

The following behavioural characteristics describe activities that can take place outside or indoors, or result in an attempt to go outside. It is undeniable, however, that the type and location of the behaviour will influence whether the actions are judged to be evidence of wandering or not (Albert, 1992; Sayer, 1994):

- pottering with purpose (busying themselves);
- following behaviour (walking behind or hovering around others);
- apparently aimless walking;
- pacing/restless movement;
- comfortable behaviour (pursuing personal habits);
- comfortable remnants (pursuing tasks from the past);
- trailing/tracking a significant other (clinging to a carer);
- searching for their past (going home, going to work, seeking children);
- attachment behaviour (when apart, seeking the proximity of a person or place that represents security);
- over-appropriate behaviour;

- exit behaviour (persistent efforts to 'get out' or 'get away');
- place disorientation (getting lost within a building);
- walking with risk toward an appropriate goal;
- appropriate goal, inappropriate time.

Confusion: A Reality Nevertheless

The essence of most people's understanding of dementia is that the person is confused. Yet the term 'confusion' encompasses a vast range of behaviours which only have in common the observation that others find them puzzling and inappropriate. Thus, usage itself can be confusing. In fact, Lishman (1987) defines confusion not in terms of actions, but as 'the inability to think with one's customary clarity and coherence'. However, as we infer a person's reasoning from the way they act, it can be more effective to assess whether they are confused or otherwise by directly assessing their behaviour, rather than speculating over thought processes. Unfortunately, there is no agreement as to what actions constitute confusion. People are said to be confused if they are restless, uncooperative, forgetful or disoriented. I was told somebody was confused when no one could understand what they were saying.

I distinguish confusion from actions that implicate error (for example, placing objects in the 'wrong' place), poor judgement (for example, putting flammable items on the cooker; drinking from the washing-up bowl), disorientation (for example, lost and bewildered) and hallucinations and delusions typical of psychosis. Thus, the following behavioural definition excludes mistake, misjudgement, 'not knowing' and psychotic phenomena. Alternative definitions are not wrong, but have simply adopted a different psychobehavioural framework.

Behavioural Definition

Confusion is the reporting of information or living of experience that represents a reality discordant to our own.

Behavioural Characteristics
Behavioural characteristics include the following:

- knowing deceased parents or partners to be alive;
- demanding to go to work;

- wanting to find or care for their young children;
- leaving home to go 'home';
- talking to strangers or professional carers as if they are 'loved ones';
- knowing partners to be parents, and adult children to be partners;
- acting inappropriately to context (for example, knowing themselves to be at work, when they are at day care).

The case of Mrs M (pp69–70) illustrates the nature of confusion. It also reveals that confusion cannot be interpreted solely as a cognitive phenomenon, for to do so is to neglect the subjective tone of dementia, a theme that will be developed in Chapter 4 and explored throughout our understanding of challenging behaviour.

Conclusion

The operational definitions described in this chapter are not set in tablets of stone. They are to be used as guides for working with people who are challenging. The methodology should encourage debate on the way we are assessing and reporting the actions of our patients and clients. Erroneous labelling or considered descriptions? Furthermore, if this discussion has challenged some of the terms used to define the syndrome of dementia, then what legitimacy can be preferred on such labels as s(he) is 'uncooperative', 'difficult', 'demanding', 'annoying', 'manipulative', 'disruptive' or 'lazy', or observations such as 'attention-seeking', 'interferes with other people's possessions' or 'objectionable to others'. What do they mean, what do they convey? I suggest little of value.

Many challenging behaviours, however, defy acceptable categorisation. Other terms cover such a range of disparate actions that the labels do not lend themselves to agreed behavioural definitions. In these instances labelling should be dispensed with, and in its place the nature of behaviour should be illuminated through detailed descriptions of actual conduct. In other words, immediate reference is made to the behavioural characteristics. As mentioned earlier, describing 'what the behaviour looks like' is known as *pinpointing*. In other words, we pinpoint precisely what a person does. Such detailed descriptions leave little room for misunderstanding, and thereby enable the practice of meaningful assessment. There are undeniable benefits to the culture of care when pinpointing informs the process of assessment, reporting and care planning. Behaviours will have been reliably observed and communicated; care plans and intervention will have been formulated on the basis of accurate information.

While those who spend most time with clients have the best opportunity to pinpoint precise behaviours, familiarity can sometimes lead to a significant difficulty: we can be so familiar with a person that we may overlook important features of their behaviour. It is sometimes difficult to stand back and look objectively at what they do. Instead we may 'see' what we expect to see.

Hence, pinpointing is a skill that requires practice. To assess accurately, we need to become objective, observe carefully, and avoid the temptation to employ vague and ill-defined labels indiscriminately.

CHAPTER 3
The 'Medical Disease' Model of Dementia

AS WE HAVE SEEN, ASSESSMENT OF BEHAVIOUR in dementia is dedicated to the accurate description of performance deficits (what a person is no longer able to do) and excesses (what a person has started to do). It is not a procedure designed to establish cause. Yet cognitive and behavioural assessment is frequently employed as if it is a diagnostic methodology (see p23). The process of assessment invariably falls victim to an unwelcome perversion of purpose: the observation of dysfunctional behaviour is automatically reduced to a neurobiological simplification that reflects the prevailing dominance of the 'medical disease' model of dementia.

Dementia is traditionally defined in terms of neurological changes in the cerebral cortex. The biomedical model assumes a causal relationship between neuropathology and dementia that fails to acknowledge the complexity of the human experience in dementia. Thus, it is an impoverished framework for an understanding of challenging behaviour. Just because we possess indirect evidence of pathology in the brain, this is not sufficient explanation for the incompetence and challenging actions observed in dementia. For too long the care of people with dementia has been dominated by the despair and negativity that seeps from a disease model that views the deteriorating profile of behaviour solely in terms of progressive neurological destruction. This has produced a culture of care that is little more than 'warehousing'; that is, meeting the basic physical needs of a person and making them as comfortable as possible (Sixsmith *et al,* 1993).

Although the underlying neuropathology eventually determines entry to a degrading incapacity, prior to the state of total incoherence and dependency psychogenic and environmental factors influence the rate and pattern of behavioural change. Environmental and psychological factors do not cause dementia, but they provide explanations for the individual behavioural consequences of the presumptive disease. Consequently, they challenge the determinism and pessimism that pervade the accepted 'medical disease' model.

To argue for the inclusion of psychosocial factors in our understanding of dementia is not to dismiss the role of neurogenic factors in the genesis of challenging behaviour. It would be a pointless exercise to replace the limited analysis of the biomedical model with imbalanced explanation and ill-founded expectation, such as that to be found in Feil (1992). Challenging behaviour may not only be secondary to the generalised impairments of memory, recognition, orientation and reasoning observed in Alzheimer's disease (see Box 3.1); there is the possibility that it may be the direct result of structural brain lesions or the degeneration of specific neurotransmitter systems.

Box 3.1 Alzheimer's disease (AD)

Named after Alois Alzheimer, the German physician who first identified this neurological disease of the cerebral cortex in 1907, this it is the most common form of dementia, accounting for at least 50 per cent of cases. Definite diagnosis can only be determined after death. AD sometimes appears in middle age (early-onset dementia, EOD), but most often it occurs after the age of 70 (late-onset dementia, LOD).

AD is progressive, irreversible and pursues an insidious unremitting course over a number of years. Dysfunction usually begins with mild memory problems, poor concentration, word-finding difficulties and impaired reasoning. These symptoms keep increasing in frequency and severity until memories are forgotten, disorientation reigns and communication fails. Eventually cognitive abilities are so severely impaired that the person becomes fully dependent upon others.

The decrease in brain cell numbers in the suprachiasmatic nucleus observed in Alzheimer's disease (Swaab *et al*, 1985) may be an explanation for excessive walking at night (Hope & Fairburn, 1990) and the increase in movement observed in the latter part of the day (the 'sundowning' phenomenon). This nucleus appears to be involved in the organisation of the sleep–wake cycle, so, as dementia progresses complete disorganisation of the rhythm of daily life occurs. Changes in brain structure have also been associated with dysfunctional walking. De Leon *et al* (1984) established an association between parietal lobe pathology and wandering. Using CT (computed tomography) data from patients with a clinical diagnosis of Alzheimer's disease, Burns *et al* (1990c) correlated wandering with increased size of the Sylvanian fissure.

Decreased levels of 5-hydroxytryptamine (5-HT or serotonin) may be implicated in aggressive behaviour that appears not to be situation-specific (Ware *et al*, 1990; Patel & Hope, 1993). There is evidence of 5-HT dysfunction in Alzheimer's disease (Bowen *et al*, 1983) and, in a small retrospective study, Palmer *et al* (1988) established an association between aggressive behaviour and 5-HT reduction. It is unlikely, however, that any simple relationship between 5-HT levels and aggressive behaviour will emerge (Patel & Hope, 1993). Temporal lobe atrophy has been correlated with aggressive behaviour in Alzheimer's disease (Burns *et al*, 1990c), while frontal-lobe pathology is associated with both aggression and abnormal sexual behaviour (Lishman, 1987; Miller *et al*, 1997). Frontal lesions can result in a destruction of the mechanisms which underlie self-control. As a result, basic impulses are released by the damage. This is of particular significance in cases of fronto-temporal dementia (See Box 3.2). A characteristic feature of Pick's disease is a Klüver-Bucy-like syndrome characterised by hypersexuality, meaningless tactile searching and indiscriminate eating.

Box 3.2 Fronto-temporal dementia (FTD)

This is dementia that is associated with cellular disease of the frontal and temporal lobes of the cerebral cortex. The prevalence of FTD has been estimated at approximately 10 per cent. In a minority of cases, FTD involves cellular degeneration, known as Pick's disease. FTD is observed as both an early and late onset syndrome, although Pick's disease is most often seen between the ages of 50 and 60 years.

The clinical features of FTD are characterised by a slow and insidious onset involving, predominantly, personality, emotion and judgement. There is a lack of initiative, indifference and neglect of responsibilities. Others may become restless, impulsive and overtly disinhibited. Obsessive-compulsive behaviour is common. In the early stages, personality and behavioural change outweigh specific cognitive symptoms. As years pass, and the disease progresses, language is affected and FTD conforms to the classical picture of Alzheimer's disease.

Burns *et al* (1990c) found that hyperorality (putting objects, other than food, in the mouth) was associated with widening of the third ventricle and atrophy of the frontal, parietal and occipital lobes. A study by Trinkle *et al* (1992) examined the related disorder of abnormal eating behaviour and failed to support these earlier findings. It did, however, support a proposal by Fairburn & Hope (1988) and Hope *et al,* (1989) that cerebral pathology damages the normal mechanism of food intake and is therefore the most likely supposition for the existence of eating abnormalities in dementia. Morley & Silver (1988) report that decreases in norepinephrine and neuro-peptide Y may be implicated in the most common change in eating behaviour in dementia, namely a decrease in the amount eaten and weight loss. As noted in the previous chapter, a significant problem with the data on eating abnormalities is that diverse oral behaviours, such as eating faeces (Ghaziuddin & McDonald, 1985), eating inappropriate foods, examining objects with the lips (Morris, *et al,* 1989), placing objects in the mouth, eating very quickly and stuffing food in the mouth (Burns *et al,* 1990c), altered food choice and a change in the mechanics of eating (Trinkle *et al,* 1992), have been aggregated to form a single category of dysfunction. This in turn limits the neuropathological conclusions that can be drawn.

Specific neuropsychological deficits observed in dementia (see Holden, 1990a; 1995) and most clearly demonstrated in vascular dementia (also known as multi-infarct dementia, see Box 3.3) are associated with challenging behaviour. Aggressive conduct has been associated with aphasia (Welsh *et al*, 1996). Eastley & Wilcock (1997) noted that aggressive behaviour occurs in approximately 20 per cent of cases of Alzheimer's disease and is associated with male gender and apraxia. Moniz-Cook *et al* (1999) describe the contribution of neuropsychological deficits to a number of 'resistance' and disruptive behaviours. Holden (1990a) illustrates how behaviours that are experienced as perplexing and challenging may be poorly understood unless reference is made to the behavioural consequences of apraxia, agnosia, perseveration and other neuropsychological decrements.

Box 3.3 Vascular dementia (VD)

Vascular dementia, also known as multi-infarct dementia, follows a series of strokes, or infarcts, when a loss of blood flow damages specific areas of the brain. The stroke may be 'silent', being so small as to pass unnoticed. Hence the stroke is often referred to as a 'strokelet'. After several 'strokelets', sufficient brain tissue may be destroyed to result in dementia. VD accounts for about 20 per cent of dementia and is generally observed in the seventh and eighth decades of life.

VD is a remitting dementia characterised by an abrupt onset. The course is typically that of a series of small strokes, which vary in frequency, intensity and location. They cause episodes of disorientation and loss of specific cognitive function. After the infarct there is usually limited clinical improvement until the next episode. As parts of the brain may be spared, or are yet to be affected by stroke, the cognitive picture is patchy and inconsistent. Eventually, after a succession of infarcts, there is less and less recovery, until by a process of 'stepwise' deterioration, dementia as widespread as Alzheimer's disease develops.

Overall, despite the dominance of what Kitwood (1989) refers to as the 'standard paradigm', a review of the data in support of the basic premise of a causal relationship between neuropathology and specific behavioural disturbance yields an unclear picture of equivocal findings.

As Hope & Patel (1993) conclude, 'little is known at present of the relationship between behaviour change and brain damage in dementia'.

Any attempt to establish the aetiology of challenging behaviour needs also to consider the psychiatric features of dementia (Haddad & Benbow, 1993b). Burns *et al,* (1990a) showed that 16 per cent of their subjects with Alzheimer's disease had delusions, the most common content concerning theft and suspicion. A further 20 per cent had experienced persecutory ideation short of delusions since the onset of dementia. Studies of multi-infarct dementia and Alzheimer's disease have reported rates for delusions of 37 per cent (Berrios & Brook, 1985), 21 per cent (Reisberg *et al,* 1987) and 31 per cent (Rubin *et al,* 1988). Cummings (1985) concluded that delusions were particularly common in subcortical dementia (see Box 3.4).

Box 3.4 Subcortical dementia

Subcortical dementia refers to the neuropsychological and behavioural symptoms of degenerative disorders involving, primarily, subcortical structures. The most common of these disorders – Parkinson's disease, Huntington's disease and progressive supranuclear palsy – can occur, however, without obvious cognitive deficits.

When dementia does arise, despite different aetiologies and certain unique neuropsychological signs, there are similarities in the pattern of spared and impaired functions. Subcortical dementia is characterised by poor concentration, apathy, low mood, forgetfulness, impaired conceptual thought, slowness of mental processing and an associated motor disorder. Symptoms of aphasia, agnosia and apraxia, the classical signs of cortical damage, are typically absent.

In the early stages of subcortical dementia, deficits show up as 'diminished efficiency' in thought and action. Cognitive decline progresses slowly and may be related to disease characteristics and duration.

Burns *et al,* (1990b) documented visual hallucinations in 13 per cent of their sample and auditory hallucinations in 10 per cent, with 30 per cent having misidentification syndromes (for example, believing people to be in the house, misidentification of mirror image, misidentification of television). In studies of Alzheimer's disease, rates of 12 per cent have been reported by Reisberg et al, (1987) for visual hallucinations, and 28 per cent by Merriam et al, (1988) for either visual or auditory hallucinations. The clinical syndrome associated with dementia of the Lewy body type (see Box 3.5) features visual and auditory hallucinations accompanied by secondary paranoid delusions (Byrne et al, 1989; Birkett et al, 1992). These psychiatric symptoms are regarded by many as a defining characteristic of the disease. McKeith et al, (1992) reported visual hallucinations and delusions in 80 per cent of their cases of Lewy body-type dementia.

Box 3.5 Dementia with Lewy bodies (DLB)

In 1912 Frederic Lewy described lesions found in the brains of people suffering from Parkinson's disease. These became known as Lewy bodies. During the 1980s, a dementia was identified at post-mortem that was found to have Lewy bodies present in the cerebral cortex. A range of terms have been proposed to describe this pathology, although today it is commonly referred to as dementia with Lewy bodies (DLB). The prevalence of DLB has been estimated to be between 15 and 25 per cent.

DLB is characterised by fluctuating cognitive impairment affecting both memory and higher cortical functions. The fluctuations are pronounced, with both episodic dementia and lucid intervals. Psychiatric symptoms are common with many cases reporting visual and/or auditory hallucinations, which are usually accompanied by paranoid delusions. People also suffer from movement disorder and falls, often typical of mild Parkinsonism. The neuropathology progresses to an end stage of severe dementia.

The prevalence of psychotic phenomena may vary with the severity of cognitive impairment, but the evidence is conflicting (Patel & Hope, 1993). A possible reason for the equivocal findings is that cognitive dysfunction can make identification of both delusions and hallucinations problematic.

Placing these psychiatric phenomena in the context of challenging behaviour, Haddad & Benbow (1993b) consider how thought and perceptual disorder may lead to 'sexual problems', while Patel & Hope

(1993) note that aggressive behaviour is sometimes directly related to paranoid delusions and hallucinations. Deutsch *et al,* (1991) found a direct relationship between persecutory delusions and hallucinations and physical aggression in dementia. An investigation into the nature of wandering reported a tendency for patients who attempt to leave secure settings to have psychotic symptoms of a paranoid type (McShane, 1994).

Finally, biological factors, independent of dementia, can also disrupt brain function and generate challenging behaviour. O'Connor (1987) concluded that in more than half the cases of behavioural disturbance in dementia, the behaviour was related to disease other than the cerebral disease itself. Delirium can result in the appearance of aggressive behaviour (Granacher, 1982; Thomas, 1988) and, as Haddad & Benbow (1993b) note, can be a precipitant of inappropriate sexual conduct. Sensory deprivation arising from visual and auditory handicaps may exacerbate memory failure and perceptual dysfunction to produce a heightened potential for behavioural disturbance. More recently, Horowitz (1997) has described the relationship between visual impairment and disruptive behaviours among nursing home residents. Moniz-Cook *et al,* (1999) report the case of a woman with dementia whose noisemaking became intolerable as her eyesight failed. Most obviously, toileting difficulties attributed to a person's dementia may be the product, directly or indirectly, of physical disability, sensory impairment, medication or localised disorder (for example, urinary tract infection, constipation, prostate disease). One must also acknowledge the potential for adverse drug reactions. Benzodiazepines and levodopa may precipitate sexual acting out (Haddad & Benbow, 1993b), neuroleptics may worsen behavioural disturbance through the pathway of delirium, while benzodiazepines may also directly cause aggressive behaviour (Patel & Hope, 1993).

CHAPTER 4

A Person with Dementia

T HE MEDICAL MODEL IS PERSUASIVE, and dominates our thinking on dementia. It is an example of biological reductionism that explains dementia in terms of:

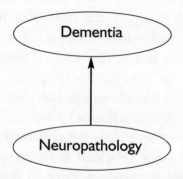

Or, as Kitwood (1989) expressed this linear causal relationship: 'x → neuropathic change → dementia', where 'x' is a causal disease which may be known or unknown. The symptoms we identify as dementia are viewed as the direct consequence of the neuropathic destruction which has been caused by this disease entity.

This standard paradigm account of dementia is 'instantly recognisable to professionals involved in dementia care and it forms the basis of the public image' of dementia (Morton, 1999). An educational leaflet published by the Alzheimer's Disease Society (1995) clearly illustrates the extent to which the medical model holds sway in the field: 'Alzheimer's disease is a physical condition. The mental and emotional symptoms are a direct result of a set of catastrophic changes in the brain that lead to the death of the brain cells.' The consequence of this view is that there is no need to address the psychological, biographical and interpersonal context within which the disease occurs. In essence there is no room for 'the person'.

Difficulties for the Standard Paradigm

A critical examination of the biomedical interpretation of dementia reveals that the assumption of an exclusive causal relationship between neuropathology on the one hand and dementia on the other is unjustified.

Post-Mortem Examination Data

A key criterion of a disease is that 'distinct pathological features be present in all cases where the symptoms appear, and in none of the cases where they do not' (Kitwood, 1997). Alzheimer's disease and vascular dementia, for example, do not meet this key criterion. Researchers have identified that clinical measures of dementia severity do not correlate well with the extent and type of neuropathic change found at post-mortem (for example, Terry, 1992). Kitwood (1989) estimates that the correlations leave 'some 80 % of the variance unexplained in moderate or severe dementia'.

Clinical Variability

Until the final stage of total incoherent dependency no two people with dementia are alike. Some are known as 'pleasantly confused' (although the pertinent question to address is, pleasant for whom?), a trouble to nobody; others display a range of challenging and demanding behaviours; some appear tormented and perplexed; the rest present as passive, withdrawn and seemingly indifferent. If the signs and symptoms of dementia are the direct result of the brain pathology, why are they not all compliant and quiet, or all noisy and aggressive? How is it that, on the path to abject incompetence and total disengagement, some maintain their daily living skills far longer than others. Why is it that some present with excellent social facades, although many do not? Once we move beyond the narrow cognitive parameters of dementia, in other words considering not only changes in memory, thinking and language, but also daily living skills, social behaviour and emotion, we notice great individual differences (for example, Magai *et al*, 1997) that are not easily accommodated within the medical model.

Catastrophic Decline

A dementing man living at home, known as 'pleasantly confused', is admitted to a respite unit when his caring wife is taken unwell. Within 24 hours of his arrival the daily diary of care resonates with the terms 'disoriented', 'aggressive', 'a wanderer' and 'incontinent'. Symptoms of dementia? A sudden, unexpected and atypical worsening of this man's neuropathological state? Or the struggles of a man who, while trying to find the toilet in an unfamiliar environment, inadvertently walked into another person's bedroom ('an aggressive confrontation'); who unknowingly took a wrong turning and ended up outside the building aimlessly walking around ('wandering'); and who never reached the toilet in time, anyhow ('incontinent'). Clearly, the acute appearance of these 'symptoms of dementia', has less to do with neurodegeneration and more to do with the context of dementia. The experience of dysfunctional levels of stress at such times has prompted Kitwood (1997) to consider also a 'stress hypothesis' of cognitive decline.

Rementia

'Under certain circumstances sufferers from Alzheimer's disease who had, apparently, gone far down the path of behavioural and cognitive impairment, can regain some of their lost faculties' (Kitwood, 1989). The phenomenon of 'rementia', wherein moderate recoveries of orientation, continence, communication and simple task competence are observed, does not represent a permanent restoration of powers. Neuropathological deterioration will ensure entry to a state of total incompetence. Yet, on the way, meaningful times of improved function, to the benefit of all, would have been achieved. In the realms of challenging behaviour and distressed emotion, however, lasting resolution is seen. Sixsmith *et al*, (1993) demonstrated in supportive, person-centred residential settings notable, albeit temporary, improvements in cognitive and functional abilities, as well as a reduction in social disturbance. That the greater improvement was identified with people who had been labelled as 'management problems' ('aggressive or anti-social patterns of behaviour, chronic anxiety and restlessness') provides compelling evidence that challenging behaviour cannot be adequately explained solely within the parameters of neurological disease.

These phenomena clearly reveal that psychological and social factors exercise powerful effects on the course of a dementing illness. A biomedical paradigm which interprets dementia solely as the consequence of brain-cell death cannot adequately account for much which is observed and known about the presentation and progression of dementia.

Why Does the Medical Model Continue to Dominate?

The biomedical framework of dementia continues to hold sway for no single reason. A complex interaction of factors serves to weave a fabric that successfully clothes the standard paradigm with credibility and authority which, at best, it only partially deserves.

The dominance of the disease model observed in general medicine understandably permeates the world of neuropathology and dementia care. Throughout this century, the discovery of neurological correlates with specific dementia profiles (for example, Alzheimer, 1907; Pick, 1904; Hachinski et al, 1974; Byrne et al, 1989), along with increasingly sophisticated methods of neurological investigation, for example radiological examinations such as computed tomography (CT) and multi-resonance imaging (MRI) encouraged a biotechnical framing of dementia. Such diagnostic explanations are straightforward and seductive in their simplicity ('A' causes 'B').

A neurological framework also enables a comforting 'no-blame' culture of care. If we regard the signs of dementia – the dependency, the intrusive, demanding behaviours – as the direct product of changes within the brain, the nature of care actions is of little consequence. As the person with dementia deteriorates and presents us with challenging conduct, we in the process can absolve ourselves of responsibility. This not only frees 'devoted and dog-tired' family supporters from the knowledge that they may be playing a role in the genesis of unwanted behaviour, it also allows the inadequate human and material resourcing of dementia care. If behaviour in dementia is interpreted as the direct product of neuropathology, rather than being seen as inextricably related to a person's life experience, issues of service quality and psychological care can be at best relegated to a subordinate status, or at worst disregarded.

Potentially, the most significant factor underpinning our belief that we can reduce our understanding of dementia to neuropathology, and thereby neglect the fact that we work with people who have dementia, people who are struggling to survive and communicate, is our dread of dementia. We must address the phenomenon of the *social distance,* the distance we place between ourselves and any group of people we fear, or feel threatened by. This distance is barren land, yet fertile ground for the creation of myths, stereotypes and prejudice. As we never get close to these people, we do not, cannot know them. Hence we can make up any stories we wish, promote any beliefs we want, with little prospect of their ever being challenged and contradicted.

To work with those who are dementing is disconcerting. I well remember my first day on the 'psychogeriatric unit': the sense of distaste and foreboding; the noise, the smell of human excrement; the disquiet of being faced with the strangeness of it all; the meaningless speech, the bizarre acts, their intimidating social presence; mysterious, unpredictable behaviour banished behind high walls and locked doors; no means of communication or reasoning with ... what? Surely not people. The grotesque tragedy that had befallen them must at least have saved them from suffering such degradation. Does not the medical model talk of signs and symptoms? There is no reference to the person; no talk of survival, anguish or torment. We can draw comfort from the knowledge that dementia is such a terrible affliction 'it destroys the person, but forgets to take the body away'. Are we not encouraged in this conviction by the words often spoken by relatives? How often do we hear husbands and wives, sons and daughters say, 'That's not my father'; 'If you had known my mother'; 'My John, he was a lovely man, he never would ...'. Box 4.1 captures the sense of loss experience by a daughter whose mother appeared to be a woman transformed.

Box 4.1

… mother was a pristine housekeeper and one of her great rituals was to lay a beautiful table at mealtimes. One day, my father noticed that she couldn't lay a knife, spoon and fork in the right order any more. She was only 54, but it was the beginning of Alzheimer's.

Each time I came home, she was less and less like my mother. Sometimes she didn't know me. She could be quite violent at times and would run out of the house with no clothes on. (The words of a loving daughter, *Daily Telegraph*, 1 April 1998)

In other words those with dementia act in ways so diametrically opposed to the way they used to be, it gives others the ammunition they require to argue understandably, that, 'For all the intimate familiarity of that face and body, I did not feel his presence beside me, only his absence' (Morris, 1995).

Their behaviour, however, is so changed, so bizarre it not only confirms the belief that they are not the person they used to be, but their conduct is so very different from our own they tragically acquire the status of a non-person. A process of objectification commences whereby the person is less regarded as a sentient being, and is seen instead as being little more than an aggregate of symptoms. The person is lost, and feelings of resentment, anger, even amusement, can be grounded in the belief that it is the disease that puzzles and disgusts us, not my father, mother, husband, wife … Thus the person is not seen as simply being changed from their previous self, they, the living embodiment of all they have ever been, is considered to have been taken from us.

How can we perpetuate this myth? Well, the social distance enables us to do so, for we never cross the divide to get to know them as people – really know them, not just the knowledge of scant demographic data, for this is not knowing somebody. That is not appreciating who they are. We need to know about people who act differently from us, but with whom we have much in common. To achieve this we need to face *our* anxieties and expend time and energy communicating with those who are difficult to see. Yet is this not a fruitless exercise? Are not their ramblings reduced to confusion, delusion and confabulation? So why devote effort to such a pointless, unrewarding pursuit? Within the biomedical framework of understanding, this is a question to be expected. However, if time is devoted reaching out to somebody with dementia, listening to them, appreciating their needs, feeling their suffering, understanding their ways, we are compelled to accept that a person with dementia is unquestionably that: a person. They have not departed.

Yet knowing somebody with dementia is a double-edged sword. For not only do we identify who they remain, we also establish who they once were, a person like us in every way. This makes us feel very uncomfortable, for, if 30 years ago they were like us, then, 30 years from now, we could be like them. And nobody wishes to dement. We retreat across the social distance and from our detached perspective, armed with and supported by the 'standard paradigm', argue not only that a person with dementia is so fundamentally different from ourselves that they cease to be a member of the human constituency, but that they were always different. In years past, they must have been quirky, eccentric, disreputable, never truly like those around them. Maybe they were always absent-minded, just managing to muddle through. Possibly the differences were subtle and slight, but there would have been some characteristic that marked them out from the rest. Maybe it was their lifestyle, or an unsavoury habit. Whatever the distinguishing feature, it is of little consequence, for we are as pure as the driven snow, and as competent as they come, so of course we will never dement. The social distance enables us to know it will not be us roaming around lost, with clothes soiled, screaming out, demanding to know where our children are. It will always be that person known by the name of 'somebody else'.

The consequences for dementia care can be dire. Care practice is likely to be task-driven, for how can it be otherwise? There is no person to relate to. Care tasks will ensure physical welfare and bodily comfort, but contribute little else. I have been privileged to observe quality care settings, but I have also come across care practice that is testimony to the 'warehousing' culture of care: dementia care units where there are low levels of social contact and little effort to engage residents in activities. Staff provide them with food and basic physical care, but little else. Over 80 per cent of the time, residents are either socially uninvolved or dozing. But is it so surprising that such little time is spent listening, talking and being with them? For if the person is lost, what is the point; where is the motivation to be found? Not only will the focus of care be task-driven, these tasks will be practised mechanically. People will be dressed, undressed, toileted, washed and bathed with little thought about what it is like to be in receipt of such intimate care. With such insensitivity, it is not surprising that residents resist and fail to co-operate. Such unco-operativeness may be interpreted as aggressive resistance, and ultimately degraded to the status of a symptom of dementia. There is no awareness of a person struggling to understand and survive behind a barrier of dementia (see Box 4.2).

Box 4.2 The embarrassment of Patrick

Patrick was referred to me because of 'deliberate incontinence'. He was unable to toilet himself, so he was on a three-hourly toileting programme. Yet only rarely would he co-operate and use the toilet. Instead, on being returned to his chair, he would soon after deliberately wet himself. His sons would protest that this was not their father. He had been such a proud and dignified man. Staff were seeing his behaviour in terms of attention seeking, manipulation and, as they regularly had to change him, a sexual problem.

The practice was for two members of staff to accompany Patrick to the toilet. Having entered the cubicle they would help him adjust his clothing and then wait beside him – on most occasions talking to each other! Is it any wonder he rarely performed? For him, his toileting had truly become a social event. The presence of the staff members was inhibiting, yet he had been cued in to the need to urinate. On his return to his chair, he was compelled to urinate. The care actions of the staff were a reflection of a disregard for *a person* with dementia.

The solution was both obvious and effective. Having positioned Patrick in the toilet and adjusted his clothing, they let him be, standing outside the door, and respecting his need for privacy and self-respect. As expected, on being left alone he would urinate appropriately. Acknowledging the person and *disregarding the dementia*, led to rementia.

Person First, Dementia Second

People are a rich tapestry of needs and preferences, hurts and fears, doubts and insecurities, strengths and weaknesses, likes and dislikes, emotions and habits. 'Unfortunately, this inner world is often denied to people with dementia' (Stokes, 1995b). Yet it is not, and never can be, the case that, on receipt of a 'diagnosis' of dementia, one acquires a label and discards one's unique individuality. As Stokes (ibid) describes, the destruction of known 'personality' is a gradual, uneven process destined to take a number of years. With the passage of time motivations will be distorted and disfigured and the person will be slowly submerged by the disease. However, understanding the reasons for challenging behaviour must always incorporate an appreciation of a person's biography and unique psychology (see Bailey *et al*, 1998; Moniz-Cook *et al*, 1999). As many others have observed, Bell & McGregor (1995) reported that people with dementia retain 'the basic core characteristics that made them the person they always were'. The longer I work with those who are dementing, the more I am impressed by their uniqueness, their struggles and our tendency to misunderstand and blame: never more so than in the case of Mrs S (Stokes, 1995b).

Case Study: Mrs S
Client: Mrs S, aged 75 years
Diagnosis: Probable Alzheimer's disease
History: Lives alone. Well supported by two caring daughters.

Presenting problem: Profoundly forgetful for everyday and current experiences, but excellent social facade. Over past three months has shown risky behaviours within the home (for example, throwing sugar on her artificial flame effect gas fire), worsening disorientation (she would be seen in her garden in the early hours of the morning inappropriately dressed) and impoverished speech content characterised by anomia (word-finding difficulty). Intact or minimally altered personal hygiene skills.

Action: Admission to an ESMI (elderly severely mentally infirm) unit to live alongside 11 people with advanced dementia.

Outcomes
1 During first week regularly found to be wet while walking around unit, as well as soiling discreetly overnight.

2 Behaviour labelled as difficult, as no interest is shown in using the two toilets available to the residents and she denies she is wet when 'confronted'. Observed to have walked in and past toilets, and to be found wet a short time later. Physical examination and laboratory investigations reveal no evidence of incontinence.

3 Mrs S does not co-operate with a toileting programme based on three-hourly 'checks and prompts'. Signs of 'aggression'.

4 Within three weeks of entry Mrs S shows evidence of depression. She says little, does little and wets herself where she sits.

Initial explanation

Deteriorating behaviour indicates advancing dementia being acted out in unfamiliar surroundings.

Revised formulation

There followed nine weeks of therapeutic inactivity during which time she was labelled as aggressive and incontinent. One day, as an aside, a distressed daughter revealed in conversation that her mother had always had an aversion to public lavatories. Her pre-morbid dread was that the toilet was not clean and hygienic. Within the limits laid down by her cognitive impairments, Mrs S was acting out an entrenched need that could not be successfully communicated.

Implemented resolution

Provision of two disposable seat cover dispensers. Effective 60 per cent of the time. When staff were unable to draw her attention to the facility Mrs S could not remember its existence and thus she would wet herself after a fruitless search for 'her' toilet. The success rate, however, was sufficient to promote satisfactory adjustment and staff tolerance.

This case demonstrates the ease with which a need that cannot be communicated can remain unacknowledged. The acting out of a need for hygiene resulted in Mrs S being labelled as incontinent. This neither recognised the origins of her difficulty nor assisted in resolving the problems presented. A significant question to ask, however, is whether the dementia caused her distaste for communal toileting arrangements, or whether it constituted a barrier that prevented Mrs S communicating her need. Obviously, it is the latter. Thus an effective methodology to adopt when working with dementia is to regard it as a barrier to seeing and understanding the person (see Figure 4.1), a barrier constructed by neurological disease and reinforced by the complicating and potentially remedial effects of ill-health, medication and disability. Yet we must not let this obstruct our path to understanding the person and the trials they face.

A biomedical interpretation fails to acknowledge that the person remains, albeit increasingly unseen. Instead whatever is seen or heard is defined as the product of the presumptive disease. In this instance, the denial of the person is facilitated by observations that Mrs S, a woman who was so concerned with personal hygiene that she refused to use public lavatories, was now seemingly content to wet and soil herself. Yet, on closer examination, she remains the same person. Her avoidance of the communal toilets and the search for her own toilet were an expression of her historical toileting need. Her cognitive impairments prevented her from appreciating the reality of her situation. Perversely, her motivation to

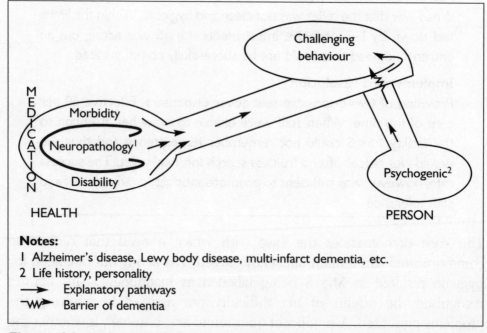

Figure 4.1 *Behavioural changes in dementia: the person (psychogenic) behind the barrier of cerebral disease (neuropathology)*

maintain personal hygiene had resulted in a profile of toileting difficulties that suggested this woman was 'lost', no longer to be acknowledged.

When the normal avenues of communication are denied, we cannot readily discover the person. Yet we cannot allow the destruction of language, memory and reasoning to be an insurmountable barrier to understanding who people with dementia are and why they do what they do. If we make contact with the person behind the barrier we are offered the opportunity to 'stand the prevailing opinion of dementia on its head and assert that much behaviour in dementia is not meaningless, but meaningful' (Stokes, 1995b).

The Person with Insight

When a person possesses insight into the frightening implications of their cognitive devastation it is easier for us to acknowledge who they are and how they feel. Maybe they never understood they were suffering from dementia, never knew the name of the responsible pathology, they simply knew something was wrong as they embarked upon a journey 'from familiarity and certainty to uncertainty; the whole underpinned by feelings of helplessness and fear' (Keady *et al*, 1995). We are sensitive to their panic and dread. In the beginning, there is little temptation to reject the person. However, as they attempt to cope, endeavour to determine their own lives, early in the process of dementia they may start to act in ways so far removed from their previous selves that the belief that they are changing, disappearing, leaving behind symptoms to be 'dealt with' begins to hold sway. We talk of 'personality change'. Unsurprisingly, the tolerance of others is stretched to the limit. A devoted husband talked of divorcing his wife if the psychiatrist could not tell him what was wrong. He described having married an intelligent and loving woman, who had turned into 'a shrew'. He used phrases such as 'a beastly person', 'a horrible piece of work', 'She was horrid'. He saw her as a 'complete stranger'. This was understandable, as his wife, still only in her early forties, was now selfish, abusive and violent. She had assaulted him and spat at him, as well as having been arrested for shoplifting.

Do the descriptions and observations of this caring man attest to personality change? Do they indicate the first signs that the person is being lost? Or do we see evidence of a person living their life as best they can, struggling with fears and self-doubt, coping with the knowledge that something is inexplicably wrong? Not only wrong, but uncontrollably so, and seemingly worsening.

Have you ever had the experience of waking in the morning, possibly when on holiday, and for a split second not knowing where you are? Welcome to dementia. Now imagine the experience is not when you are waking in the comfort and safety of a bedroom but any time, anywhere, without warning and … 'the penny doesn't drop'. How do you feel? Can you imagine standing in front of the refrigerator, not knowing whether you have just closed it or are about to open the door?

We have all had the experience of walking into a room and puzzling as to why, or racing upstairs only to ask ourselves, 'What have I come up here for?' We have all lost the thread of a conversation, forgotten somebody's name, mislaid everyday items. But what if it was to happen more and more often, with recall rarely, if ever, returning. How would you cope? What would you do? Keady *et al* (ibid) describe the challenges faced by those with early dementia, the frustrations of:

- forgetting messages,
- not being able to put names to faces,
- being unable to follow conversations,
- being unable to remember what has been done, and what has not,
- not knowing what one had planned to do, or was currently in the midst of doing,
- getting lost,
- being unable to complete tasks previously taken for granted (for example, what goes where on returning from the supermarket),
- struggling to use everyday domestic appliances,
- not finding the right words,
- feeling overwhelmed by the demands of everyday tasks,
- poor judgement and silly mistakes,
- being out of control or, worse, being seen by others to be out of control.

It is not surprising that we hear people with dementia say: 'I couldn't believe I was doing these things. I felt so stupid and didn't want to share it with anyone in case my fears were confirmed.' Keady *et al* (ibid) observed that there were 'strong motivating factors for keeping the early stages secret even from the person with whom they were living'. We enter the subjective world of defence and deception. As the person attempts to cover up, the insidious impairments of memory and thought acquire the status of dark secrets. A psychology of dementia now unfolds. In the process, the person's mechanisms of defence and chosen means of coping may convince others that personality is changing. But this is not so, it just appears so. Coping may include denial, adaptive paranoia or confabulation.

Denial
Not wishing to acknowledge the enormity of their tragedy, a person with dementia may steadfastly deny errors, failings of memory and misjudgements. To the exasperation of others, who are only too aware that something is wrong, the person refuses to countenance the prospect of mistakes and absent-mindedness.

Adaptive Paranoia
Never again will anything be lost, it will have been stolen. Items are not mislaid, others have moved them. Appointments are not forgotten, the arrangements were never made. The person accuses others, often those who are closest, in an effort to establish external cause for their own failings. The resulting suspicion and 'paranoia' is often observed by families as an early sign of 'dementia'. To psychiatrists, the sense of persecution may be misinterpreted as evidence of psychotic delusion. For the person with dementia, they just wish for peace of mind at a time of advancing chaos.

Confabulation
Severe dementia is often characterised by reports of moments from a life once lived. Ask what the person has been doing, where have they just been, and we hear a fiction: not an outrageous fiction, but an account of how life used to be lived. In the beginning, however, confabulation possesses powerful defensive qualities. Time will be lost and items mislaid, often without the person's knowledge. When confronted with their errors, when asked to account for their late arrival, the person will trawl their memories for an everyday, non-threatening explanation for their failings (see Box 4.3). The more they protest their explanation, the

more they persuade, not only others, but themselves that nothing is seriously amiss. Anxieties abate, and the person can cope. Of course, as time passes their explanations become increasingly implausible, yet, for the person, defence is their sole objective. To disagree or query will simply trigger denial or accusation. When insight goes, confabulation continues as a form of engagement when the person is prompted to explain, or is included by others in conversation.

Box 4.3 Confabulation as defence

A husband, exasperated by the increasing number of packets of fish fingers in the freezer, confronts his wife to get an explanation. Her response is that they are on special offer, so constitute a 'good buy'. In reality, she is unable to recall when shopping what is, and is not, required, so she purchases whatever she typically needs. Her explanation provides her with comfort, although for her husband tolerance continues to be challenged.

Disinclination to go Out

Is it surprising that, as memory worsens, a person with dementia wishes to stay home? For many of us, home is a place of safety and security. With a tendency to get lost or 'go blank' without warning, being out and about is a potential source of fear and dread. In contrast, being at home is reassuring. Hence shopping, visiting, or going to work may all be avoided. The person appears unadventurous, unreasonable and unreliable. Such actions not only limit risk, they are also psychologically comfortable, for they reduce the volume of evidence that there is something seriously wrong. Staying at home doing little yields only limited demonstrable evidence of impairment. However, such action is unlikely to be accompanied by honest and open explanation. An unwillingness to share fears, the determination to construct the facade of a life being lived well and the success of psychological defences will all lead to a preponderance of feeble excuse and a reluctance to talk.

Avoidance of Others

Hand-in-hand with a wish to stay home is a desire to be away from others. In part, this is because faces are not recognised, names are forgotten and the right words fail to appear. Embarrassment and frustration are compounded, however, by a tendency not only to lose the thread of the conversation but to repeat oneself. Questions are asked again, topics are raised as if for the first time. The other person can rarely disguise their puzzlement. As a consequence, it is little wonder that the person with dementia withdraws and avoids others. The wife of a patient of mine was infuriated by the insular attitude of her dementing husband. He would avoid company and occupy himself in the garden. His enjoyment of physical labour and the achievement he again found led him to be driven, if not compelled, to work hour after hour in his splendid garden. Maurice explained his embarrassment when having to talk to family and friends, how he would become anxious and bemused if he found himself faced with a group of people. As friends began to feel increasingly ill at ease, his wife became more and more isolated. She had lost not only the relationship with her husband, but her friendships. As she became increasingly resentful there was a corresponding decrease in the quality of care she could provide. Inevitably, entry to a nursing home was to follow.

Self-Centredness
Selfishness, irrational at times will surface as the person establishes routines to compensate for their fragile memory. If life is predictable then there is less need consciously to remember; you can work on 'automatic pilot'. So tasks will be carried out at certain times on certain days in specific ways, and woe betide anybody who suggests change. For if it is change, it is new, and if it is new it must be learned and that is where the problem lies. Such information is increasingly difficult to store. Hence the person comes over as inflexible, too set in their ways. Life may be so well ordered that there will be a place for everything, and everything in its place. They can reach out and there it will be. Yet it is difficult for others to live such a structured life, and this may be responsible for deteriorating relationships. There may be explosions of temper and distressing accusations as household items and possessions are innocently moved and the person with dementia reacts with anger.

A changing personality, a person lost, or a person, known and loved, struggling to cope with indescribable fear and apprehension. Would we act differently in similar circumstances? I believe not. You, as you are today, can envisage reacting in similar ways. The essence of you would not have to change to do so. Nor has the person with dementia changed, it just appears so. The frequent reports of hostility and paranoia, secrecy and denial, withdrawal and inflexibility make so much sense when placed within the context of a *person* enduring the subjective experience of dementia.

However, when insight is lost does a psychology of dementia remain? Traditionally, the answer has been no. When insight goes, it is invariably said that the worst is now behind them. We can be sensitive to the tragedy of somebody losing control and knowing their world is disintegrating, but when that knowledge goes it is so easy to lose sight of the person struggling to survive in a world of strangeness and torment. We are seduced by the medical model, protected by the social distance, and content to compile symptom checklists of cognitive deterioration, dependency and behavioural disturbance. I am convinced the person remains and if we are to achieve a true understanding of dementia, their psychology must be at the forefront of our thinking. The following says so much that is fundamental to our work: *just because the person loses insight, do not lose sight of the person.*

The Psychology of Dementia

In 1987, I began to talk of the phenomenology of dementia: the inner, subjective experience of dementia. The complexity of both the origins and presentation of challenging behaviour encouraged me to appreciate that much of what I was trying to understand was driven by the person within. They remained an 'active agent', interpreting their world and addressing their needs. As Rogers (1951) stated: 'The best vantage point for understanding behaviour is from the internal frame of reference of the individual himself.' A dementing person will select the manner of behaving which is the most effective in the light of how they interpret their experiences. What is deemed reasonable and appropriate is, however, subjective, not objective. This has profound implications for the way we relate to people with dementia. If we address their experience we gain insight into their world and appreciate the sense they are making of reality, at which point the meaningless and apparently bizarre may become meaningful and understandable.

While we can postulate the nature of their subjective reality, I do not wish to commit the error of Lao-Tse's companion, who, when hearing the Chinese philosopher talk of the joy of fishes, responded: 'But how can you know what joy is to a fish?' To which Lao-Tse replied: 'But how can you know what I know?' We cannot be arrogant and presume that we *know* the perceptions and thoughts of a person with dementia. Through observation, listening, enquiry and interpretation we can, however attempt to get close to their experience, to feel it as if it is our own, and then, it is hoped, enter their frame of reference.

True to Myself, Getting on with Life

We have acknowledged the uniqueness of the person. A person who, despite their dementia, will live their life as they see fit, addressing their habits and doing their best. Consequently, challenging behaviour can be the consequence of a 'comfortable behaviour' or a motivational response that is appropriate to the present but has been distorted by the limits of their neuropathology. 'Comfortable behaviour' is the way we are, a challenging continuation of who we have always been. It is our automatic ways, topics of conversations and daily habits. To partake in them feels right. So when I get up in the morning, I want a cup of tea, a newspaper and solitude. And that is what I will continue to want. It is appropriate and will be triggered by such phenomena as surroundings and the time of day. But now judgement is impaired, perceptions are faulty and concentration is poor. Hence the outcome may be unwelcome, exasperating and potentially invasive actions. If you also enjoy your own company first thing in the morning, need time to gather your thoughts, never wishing to have people around, how well would you cope in the social world of care, being sat in a communal lounge just moments after being taken out of bed and dressed? Could this be why you walk away or resist efforts to get you to sit down with others?

What may be seen by others as radically new may in fact not be so. It may be consistent with or represent an exaggeration of previous personal traits, the presentation of which have been altered by the disease, and are now regarded as challenging. At times, the comfortable behaviour may possess the characteristics of a remnant (see p72), yet this is only because we have inadequately resourced a person's present. Recently, I saw Florence who was causing havoc in the garden of the nursing home, as well as giving rise to serious concern for her welfare. She would stroll around the grounds gathering flowers, and then return indoors and eat them. This ceased to be perplexing when one knew of her passion for growing fruit and herbs! At the time her conduct was inappropriate, a remnant from her past. Next summer it will be an acceptable comfortable behaviour, for the garden will have been resourced to meet her needs.

Maybe the actions are evidence of motivational responses to resolve perceived practical problems or to be effective in daily life. There are stories, possibly apocryphal, of people cutting the grass with scissors, or 'mowing' the lawn with a vacuum cleaner. Many practitioners know of clients who have placed electric kettles or plastic bowls instead of saucepans on their cooker. Many efforts to toilet result in a failure of adaptive behaviour and are wrongly interpreted as incontinence. Box 4.4 provides a case illustration of adaptive behaviour which, taken at face value, can easily be dismissed as destructive conduct, yet on further examination resonates understanding.

Box 4.4 Client H, a 72-year-old man with probable Alzheimer's disease

H had slashed the new sports jacket his wife had purchased only the day before with a pair of scissors. Her interpretation was that, in retaliation for removing his favourite, albeit soiled, suit he had been deliberately malicious and destructive.

H could never settle. He would roam around the house taking little time to rest. As a result his wife would leave sandwiches in the kitchen so he could 'graze' while walking. During the course of eating, H had more than likely inadvertently squeezed the contents of a sandwich down the front of his jacket, and then lacked the intellectual capacity to successfully effect his desired course of action. He could not tell his wife of his accident because of significant speech impairment. Nor did his reasoning decrements enable him to sponge the stain. Instead he had picked up a pair of scissors and cut out the piece of cloth. Is this a man with no regard for his clothing, or a person who remains concerned about his appearance?

A Common Bond

We acknowledge a unique individual, yet this is founded on a basic premise, a fundamental that asserts that, as we are, a person with dementia remains a feeling, sentient being with whom we have more in common than that which separates us. What distinguish us are our contrasting intellectual powers. What we share are those essential needs that define our humanity, the essence of what it means to be human.

Goudie & Stokes (1989) first proposed that much challenging behaviour can be understood within the framework of poorly communicated need. While higher psychological needs acquired in maturity through the process of learning and acculturation are destined to be lost, along with their behavioural correlates, comparatively early in the disease process, basic human needs, those that originate in infancy and childhood, remain until the final state of passive incoherence. These include not only physiological needs, but also fundamental psychological needs, such as safety, sociability, curiosity and activity. This basic human psychology is not acquired in adulthood, but is instead embellished in our years of maturity. Social influences and learning experiences serve to modify the expression of need and mould behavioural patterns that result in successful resolution. Eventually, motives that at first were involved in the satisfaction of basic needs become functionally autonomous. However, with an increasing inability to communicate and act out need in a recognisable, accessible manner, behaviour in dementia is invariably interpreted as meaningless and devoid of purpose. We are observing, however, not the destruction of need itself, but a process of deconstruction that results in the loss of the learned enrichment of basic need. While ways of behaving are progressively lost, need states still energise behaviour in dementia. A state of agency remains. This does not mean, however, that actions can be predicted or readily associated with the inner world of motivation. For example, the experience of low-grade chronic pain in dementia and the need to be pain-free may present as shrieks and shouts, irritability, spiteful actions calling out for a parent, withdrawal or apparently aimless walking. As was noted long ago by Hebb (1955), needs are 'an engine but not a steering wheel'. This applies even more in dementia. The loss of enrichment does not result in a repertoire of easily recognised motivational behaviour. Instead, we observe behavioural ruin and chaos. The result is a dysfunctional and at times grotesque distortion of goal-directed communication and conduct that is acted out within, and contaminated by, the constraints of cognitive impairment. Observable 'personality' is therefore altered, sometimes out of all recognition. It is little surprise, therefore, that personality change induced by organic brain damage is included in the diagnostic criteria for dementia (WHO, 1990).

Yet personality at its most fundamental level has not changed. Yes, prevailing actions are at variance with the person once known, but these actions are an inadequate measure of the essential core of the person. An unadventurous, somewhat timid woman lived a sheltered life. Within the undemanding limits she set for herself, she was safe and content. Untroubled, she was a gentle, pleasant woman, always willing to help others. Tragically, she shows signs of early dementia. She finds herself on an assessment unit, a strange, noisy, invasive environment. Unsurprisingly, her need to be secure drives her to leave the unit. When prevented from doing so, she becomes violent. She spits at staff blocking her way. Are these actions inconsistent with her pre-morbid self; behaviour 180 degrees away from the gentle woman she used to be? Yes. But a person lost? No. She would always have acted in this manner if her need for security had been violated. It is just that having constructed a life that was without threat, she was never driven to acts of desperate self-protection. Her need for security led her to adopt a sheltered lifestyle, now it has resulted in violent acts of self-destruction.

The wife of Mr D (Stokes, 1996) struggled with her husband's enduring need to be safe, for, during the course of his dementia, it appeared he was determined to destroy the home he had once loved. He was driven, day after day, to collect rocks and large stones from his gardens and store them in neat piles in the garage. From early morning to the end of the day, he would work in the garden. Collecting his wheelbarrow and spade, he would walk to a flower bed and systematically destroy it. Flowers, shrubs and small trees were pulled out or hacked down. He would then shovel as much soil as he could into the wheelbarrow, and wheel his barrow onto the lawn where he would empty the contents. Separating the soil from the rocks and stones, he would wheel the latter to his garage. Returning to the garden he would gather up as much soil as his judgement would allow and deposit it onto the flower bed. As the weeks passed, he destroyed his gardens. Occasionally, he would vary his behaviour. Instead of wheeling his barrow onto the lawn, he would bring it into the house and empty its contents onto the carpet. The hall and lounge carpets became damp, dirty and home to a large number of bugs.

Mrs D protested, 'Why me, why us?', 'Why is he doing this to me?' Therapeutic suggestions hinged on a need to contain the problem. Sedation was regularly advised, as was removal to a secure living arrangement elsewhere. To be told her husband's behaviour was the result of dementia offered neither solace or solution.

Conversation with his wife revealed a man who had, as the years passed, become increasingly concerned about personal safety and home security. This line of conversation exposed an enduring psychological need being acted out through the lasting knowledge of a traumatic experience rooted in personal history. Years earlier, in the course of an attempted burglary, a gang of youths had thrown masonry through the window of his shop. Fifteen years on, now dementing, Mr D continued to wrestle with his enduring need to be safe. His drive for security was affected, however, by the trauma from his past. This was the psychological context for his actions. His conviction was that his home would be attacked in the same way as his shop had been. His motivation was to protect himself and his wife from such hazards. The emotions associated with the attempted robbery were no longer tempered by the passage of time, but felt with the force of the original moment, and they generated a powerful motive for action.

Mr D's devastated capacity to reason prevented him from appreciating that people rarely, if ever, attack your home with rocks and stones from the garden. Consequently, his conduct appeared bizarre, without reason. His disintegrating behavioural patterns served to obscure his psychology, rather than providing a gateway to his inner world of need and feeling. This is a common theme in dementia. Similarly, if not saying what you mean, or meaning what you say, applies to any group of people, it is those with dementia.

A person with dementia may not only act out their needs. Alternatively, they may attempt to communicate, unfortunately with little success. We hear their words, but are we listening? Five themes of life are commonly expressed. They ask for, or enquire after, their parents, children, partners, home and jobs. On the one hand, this appears to be evidence of living in the past: in other words, confusion. On the other hand, maybe the person is using words to articulate a need. It is not what they wish to say, but it is the only language that remains. They may ask for their parents. Miesen (1993) developed the hypothesis that Alzheimer's disease generates 'strangeness', which in turn activates attachment behaviour that is manifest as 'parent fixation', an expression of need that cannot be automatically dismissed as evidence of confusion, confabulation or delusion. Instead it can be seen as the communication of the need to be in the proximity of another person who provides tenderness and a sense of safety and security. As we know, parents provide without question care and love and, during troubled times they are a comforting source of protection. As people with dementia live with a 'kind of psychological pain whose persistence and intensity we can scarcely envisage' (Kitwood, 1989), they may reach out for such compassion and utter the words, 'Where's my mother' (see Box 4.5).

Box 4.5

The drive to London was a nightmare. Iris protested wildly. We were going the wrong way – she must get out – where was her mother? Screams and tears. (John Bayley, writing of his wife, Iris Murdoch, *Sunday Times*, November, 1998)

Asking to go home may represent an attempt to communicate a need to belong or be safe. A woman who asks for her children may be desperately communicating a need to be needed. Demanding to go to work may be a plea to be useful and occupied. Asking for a husband or wife suggests a need for emotional warmth, companionship or sexual intimacy. Concealed messages abound.

It is clear that an objective of clinical practice, whether through observation or effective communication, is to decipher the meaning of the words and behaviour heard and seen in dementia. If we are successful, needs are identified and met. No longer will we be party to the frustration of motivation and drives (Stokes & Goudie, 1990). In this way the person is no longer unknown and irrelevant, but rediscovered and partially restored.

Understanding increases the prospect of solution. Yet even when resolution is not possible, as the behaviour loses its mystery it can generate tolerance. For Mr D's wife, with tolerance came the potential to cope, even though the situation was basically unchanged. Actions remain challenging, but others can now appreciate that they are not living with, or caring for the shell of what went before. It is not possible to respect a symptom or to care for a disease. We can only respect and care for people. With the person restored to life, identification with their suffering occurs, compassion returns and the blaming stops.

A Time of Not Knowing
This person that we now know, unique but with whom we share so much, experiences a subjective reality that is difficult for us to comprehend, for to dement is to enter a time of 'perpetual not knowing', a state of rarely, if ever, knowing where you are, how you arrived, who others are and possibly of greatest significance, what will happen next. This is disorientation. When there is an inability to store information and learn, the unfamiliar never loses its mystery. A pervasive sense of uncertainty prevails. And this state is often experienced in a world that is unsupportive and depersonalised (Kitwood, 1990). It may be endured while living alone or in the company of people with dementia – not *other* people with dementia, for we have reached the point on the journey where insight has been lost. A person with severe dementia does not appreciate they are dementing. They do not live alongside others with dementia, sharing a 'Dunkirk spirit'. There is no bond of compatriotism founded on an awareness of mutual difficulties.

Instead, their social world is an aggregation of others who are unlike them: people who act in unpredictable, asocial and intimidating ways. Any one of them may act out, but in the absence of a capacity to retain novel information, they will forget within moments their own errors and misdemeanours. Hence, if we observe 10 adults with dementia, we see 10 dementing people. To be one of those adults is to see nine 'mad', 'bad', 'peculiar', people and yourself: you as you have always been.

A tragedy for people with dementia is that, even when they remain in the place that is most familiar to them, namely their own home, surrounded by people who know them best, their family and friends, as time passes and memory disintegrates according to the principle of Ribot's law (that which is experienced last is lost first), any vestige of security is destroyed. The familiar becomes unfamiliar, frighteningly and

67

increasingly so. Partners and children will no longer be recognised, a home ceases to be reassuring. This strangeness may leave them bewildered and agitated. A caring husband, exhausted by the endeavours of the day, eventually gets his wife to bed. As he settles down alongside her, she rails at him. For who is this man, this stranger climbing into bed with her? The image she has of her husband is of a man many years younger. This person is an unrecognisable stranger. So being true to the woman she has always been, she is driven to protect herself. Unfortunately, such behaviour also renders her an increasingly unrecognisable stranger to her husband. Mutual strangeness prevails.

For some, the subjective experience of dementia is to occupy both a world of knowing and not knowing. The neuropathological destruction of most recent memories leaves only those from the past, and it is these which constitute the foundation of a life to be lived again. Once more they will have parents, young children and jobs to go to. It is not that they bring their past into the present, the past is all there is. Yet where are these loves ones? Why are they not where they should be? Curiosity, if not torment generates a determination to search. We see confusion, they experience frustration and yearning. The case of Mrs M (Box 4.6) illustrates that a person with dementia acquires a concept of self based, not on what they do or who we know them to be, but on who they *know* themselves to be, a knowledge based on known features of their history, a time passed, but again restored to the 'here and now'. It is not that they experience a chronologically determined unfolding of historical events, re-experiencing their lives as lived. Instead, their acting out of personal history encompasses over-learned ways of being and milestones and themes (parenthood, work, home, parents and partners) of emotional significance. It is these experiences and aspects of self that are most resistant to dementia. The vividness of the experience, the emotional force of the moment, the number of times you think about it result in the biochemical process of 'long-term potentiation', memories that become fixed, 'secured' and which, in dementia, constitute a world, not of belief, but of entrenched and enduring conviction. This is a past that does not simply provide a psychological context for their motivations (see the cases of Mr D, p64, Mrs O, p78 and Mrs D and the *Colour Purple*, p104), for this is their psychological reality: an appreciation of self founded not on the objective features of a situation, but on subjective awareness. This is a reality very different from our own, one that may possess little internal logic, but which is, nevertheless, a reality as meaningful to them as ours is to us.

Box 4.6 Mrs M : a case study of knowledge or belief?

A woman with early-onset dementia (she was only 51-years-old), Mrs M struggled with her inability to cope with memory impairment. She found difficulty in storing information that was new, on-going or recent. Her prospective memory (memory of things you have to do in the future) often let her down.

As a consequence, her conduct was characterised by disorientation, error and muddle. Understandably, she was anxious and fearful. She avoided other people, stayed within the safety of her own home and accused others to conceal her own mistakes. She slowly lost insight. As the months progressed, she was increasingly unreliable and unpredictable. She was unable to pursue her career, and so took early retirement on the grounds of ill-health.

On the first day of her retirement, when she awoke, where did she go? To work. Mrs M cannot store information; this is the essence of her dementia and thus she has no recall of yesterday's events: the farewells, the gifts and so on. She is, from our perspective, confused. She does not *believe* she has a job, she *knows* it. It is a given. She has worked for years, it is an unquestionable, inviolable 'fact'. As the weeks and months pass, she frequently troubles others as she attempts to leave home to go to work, protests as others prevent her from leaving, gets lost if she successfully finds herself outside. Her reality is different from ours, but it is nevertheless as meaningful to her as ours is to us.

Yet Ribot's law gradually and remorselessly exercises its effect: the destructive process of most recently *established* memories. As time passes, she is more inclined on awaking to seek her young children, who need to go to school. She does not believe she is a mother, she knows it. Her career has not happened. There has been no passage of time. She knows she has young children. Her desperate searching and pleading is founded, not on belief, but on total conviction. Have you ever lost sight of your children? Can you recall how you felt, with stomach churning, limbs weak, heart pounding, frantic? This is her experience, and this is what we label 'confusion': a term that fails to do justice to the trauma and anguish this woman is now suffering.

Why most enter a state of uncomplicated not knowing, bewildered and bemused, while others relive their past with unfailing conviction, is not known. It is difficult to suggest a neuropathological explanation for, as we have already seen, variability is difficult to accommodate within the disease model. The explanation is likely to be psychological, and potentially lies within the 'ego strength' of the individual. It could reflect a resolve borne out of a determined, controlling personality: a person who needs to know; who cannot tolerate uncertainty; or who feels ill at ease when out of control. The question, however, remains to be answered.

Another question that is often asked is, how does a person with dementia maintain their reality? How do they know they are at work when their present surroundings must be so different? When they are searching for young children, why does contemporary fashion, the design of today's cars that pass by, the technology around them not challenge and undermine their ability to hold onto a reality at variance with our own? How is it that a man always knows that every female carer who works at the day centre is his wife, when their appearances are so very different? There are no easy answers to these questions, but I believe the interrelatedness of a number of subjective phenomena contribute to our understanding.

First, never underestimate the capacity of your mind to create its own reality. All of us will take to our graves a vast catalogue of memories that give us a picture of who we are and who we have been. Some of these memories constitute *psychological 'givens'*, the themes that *you know* to be true. You know you have a home, partners, parents, children and a job. These phenomena persist throughout much, if not all, of our lives and provide the context for our experiences. When you wake up in the morning you do not run through a mental checklist to confirm these still pertain. They are incontrovertible features of your life. With an inability to retain new information and the destruction of recent and inconsequential memories, a person with dementia is anchored in a reality characterised by these enduring and emotionally significant 'facts' of life. When they awake they must be at home. If they feel ill at ease and insecure then home must be elsewhere. If it is daylight outside and they are inside, they must be at work. Or, if it is too homely, they must leave for work. If a woman is sitting watching television then the man next to her must be her husband, for it was always so. Have you ever walked past somebody you know well, because you did not expect them to be there? Maybe in dementia the opposite applies. The mind is being deceived by its own knowledge of the world.

Secondly, many memories are not adorned by the background details of the moment as lived. Recall a family holiday when you were a child, or out shopping with your mother. Remember your school days. Think about your first football match, or that memorable rock concert. Think of your first date. Do your memories resonate with a sense of being 'old fashioned' or 'out of date'? I doubt it, because what you recall is yourself and your feelings, and these are not tainted by the passage of time. But now look at photographs of these moments. Did you really wear that? Look at the cars and style of clothing. Old fashioned? Embarrassingly so? This is the explanation for our shocked expression and outbursts of laughter. For this is not how our past feels. Our *memories* are different, virtually timeless. In fact, our recall of the past is often distorted by our perceptions of today, so the backdrop to our memories is often unwittingly adorned with the trappings of current experience. Hence, *in the absence of collateral memory*, a person with dementia can easily walk down the street searching for their children or insisting they are somewhere else untroubled by the nature of their surroundings.

Third, have you ever been sitting at a table eating a meal in the company of people you do not know, who were also sitting at tables eating? Where were you? A restaurant? But did you consider the possibility you might have been in the dining room of a residential or nursing home eating your meal with fellow residents? Did you enquire of those people who you thought could be waiters, whether they were in fact care assistants? I would be concerned if you did, because why would you do so? It is *outside your experiential framework*. It is so removed from your experience and expectations of life as to play no part in your interpretation and comprehension of yourself and your world. But why should it be different for a person with dementia? With no insight, no recall of recent experience (remember the plight of Mrs M) how can we expect them to know 'our' reality? If I was to be sat on a bed one night by a young woman who started to remove my clothes, what are the chances that my actions would be tempered by a consideration that I could be a resident, and she, my keyworker? For a man with dementia, why would it be different? Why would it ever enter his frame of reference that his interpretation of her actions could be wrong? He does not know he is dementing. His actions will be guided by his experience of intimate contact with women, not by the experience of a life that he does not understand and, most significantly, is no longer living. One day, you may be sitting in a chair fiddling with a magazine while holding it upside down, repetitively turning the pages, and you will know you are reading a book on challenging behaviour in dementia, for that is what you used to do, but are you now?

Appreciating these psychological dynamics enables us to realise how easy it is to remain confused and the futility of our efforts to inform and correct. You know your reality, they know theirs. If yours is not amenable to correction, then how can theirs be?

Finally, some people with dementia appear to occupy a point mid-way between disorientation and confusion. When questioned they confabulate (this is not defence, but just an account of how life used to be lived) at other times they act out comfortable remnants associated with their history (see Box 4.7). Often these people present as untroubled. There seems little depth or emotional investment in their conduct. They do not search and demand 'to know'. Instead, they benignly live their lives. Frequently known as 'pleasantly confused' their behaviour may at times cause irritation and concern. For example, Horace, a retired electrician troubled staff greatly at the nursing home as he walked around 'fiddling' with plugs and table lamps.

Box 4.7 A bizarre symptom of dementia or a comfortable action to be understood?

A woman would spend her days making a circular motion with her hands. Sometimes this would occur while she was walking, at other times she would be quietly sitting. On occasion she would stand over a table or face a wall and perform the action. Disconcertingly she would sometimes stand in front of somebody and go through the motion of … what? A mystery. Were these bizarre, meaningless movements? The staff, familiar with her history, knew otherwise. Emily had worked for many years in the textile industry. Her job had been to feel the cloth and, if she felt a snag, she would pull it through. The actions were a testimony to her occupational self – conduct at variance with her current circumstances, no doubt, but not without meaning. Of course, if nobody had known Emily and her past, the interpretation of her behaviour might easily have led to the view that she was displaying a troublesome 'symptom' of dementia.

Conclusion

This is the subjective life of a person with dementia (see Table 4.1): a person who remains an active agent; an individual who makes decisions and initiates actions, while residing in a reality that resonates 'not knowing'; a person who, as a consequence, may be sorely misunderstood. As they live their lives, express their needs, address their problems, it is we who become equally exasperated and bemused. This puzzlement is compounded by the observation that their perceptions and motivations are transient. A fragmentation of self and experience is determined by the length of their impoverished memory span. As dementia progresses, life is little more than one disjointed fragment built on another. The failure of memory storage leads to a life increasingly lived in the immediate, a world of here and now. Motives, springs for action, are rapidly forgotten. Thus, while much behaviour in dementia is the product of motivational action, a failing capacity to retain goal-directed behaviour results in conduct that is apparently without purpose. Initially, however, there would have existed a motivated state of behaviour. Trying to explain why a person with dementia does what they do when they do it is like grasping a bar of wet soap. One moment it appears securely in your grasp, the next it is gone!

Challenging behaviour is the outcome of this chaotic, inconstant psychology:

- comfortable and adaptive behaviours that call out for knowledge of the person and an empathy for the experience of dementia;
- the communication of need through words and deeds that requires an appreciation of what it means to be human, unique but also having much in common with us all, and which demands

interventions that drive us toward the meeting of need rather than containing the consequences of not doing so;

- reliving a past with conviction and feeling, less likely to benefit from correction and reorientation, but should we instead collude, distract, ignore or, most significantly, validate the subjective truth of their experience?

The implications for assessment and analysis are clear. To allow us to understand the nature and origins of challenging behaviour the imperatives that flow from the person-centred model of dementia are the following:

- pinpointing precise descriptions of behaviour (Chapter 2),
- achieving an accurate and comprehensive medical diagnosis (Chapters 1 and 3),
- obtaining demographic information,
- acknowledgement of a person with needs common to us all (Chapters 4 and 6),
- acceptance of a unique person with a biography and personal characteristics (Chapter 4), and
- empathy for the subjective experience of dementia (Chapter 4).

Information gathering, the process of establishing both 'what' and 'why', must address all of these issues and, as we will see in the next chapter, much more besides.

Table 4.1 *The person-centred model of dementia*

We accept a person who is unique (life history, fears, joys, habits, and so on) We acknowledge a person with whom we have much in common	The subjective experience of dementia – a world of not knowing

CHAPTER 5

The Environmental Context of Dementia

NEUROPATHOLOGY IS INEXTRICABLY woven into the pattern of an individual's life history and personality, and suffered as a subjective experience. The person remains an active agent initiating, yet also *responding to* events. While they determine much from within, they are also affected by their life setting. Their environments may serve to exaggerate, potentially even create, dysfunctional behaviours. Hence, when understanding dementia, environmental circumstances and the quality of social relationships are essential components of the explanatory 'equation'. For example, the lack of privacy on most continuing-care wards for people with dementia makes 'inappropriate sexual activity in public inevitable' (Haddad & Benbow, 1993b). Inadequate building design is responsible for much misconduct that falls under the rubric of 'toileting difficulties'.

Similarly, aggressive behaviour is invariably a response to the actions of others. Meyer *et al* (1991), in a study of aggressive episodes in a population of hospitalised patients, found the vast majority of incidents were directed against others and were commonly triggered by being asked to do something. Aggressive behaviour cannot therefore be divorced from the circumstances in which it arises, and resolution is often a function of whether caregivers can adopt new ways of relating to the person with dementia.

What is the Environment?

When we consider the environment, we do not confine ourselves to the buildings within which people live ('the built environment'); we also address what is of even greater significance when understanding behaviour in dementia, namely the world of attitudes and interpersonal relationships ('the social environment'). We also distinguish between the 'situation' and 'context'. The 'situation' is the face-to-face contact between those who live with or care for a person with dementia that occurs within a specific location. The 'context' is the environmental setting within which these people live and work. In professional care settings we make reference to custom and practice, rules and regulations, the quality and availability of material and human resources, and, as has been noted by several investigators (for example Dean *et al*, 1993; Kitwood, 1997), the framework provided by the policies and management of the home to support, supervise and recognise each staff member as an individual with needs as important as those of residents. These factors exercise a profound influence over the caregiving regime. Within family care, contextual factors pertain to such issues as marital history and family dynamics. For example, a loveless marriage is not transformed into a tender, tolerant relationship simply because one of the partners develops dementia.

While it is often possible to identify situational factors involved in the causation and maintenance of challenging behaviour, wider contextual features may be of greater significance. These may create the circumstances responsible for the situational triggers and in turn may obstruct desired remedial intervention. Looking beyond a limited view of the environment, so as to take into account contextual influences, is known as 'behavioural ecology'.

The Built Environment

The built environment is the architecture, building design, interior layout, furnishings and decoration. Much of what relates to the material world is contextual, but there are always specific situational experiences. For example,

- poor lighting within a bedroom that leads to challenging misinterpretations and disorientation,

- an anonymous corridor that results in bewilderment and agitation,
- the obstruction of a door that generates frustration and noise making,
- the insecure perimeter gate that results in 'risky wandering',
- the comfortable chair that hinders movement and results in 'attention-seeking' calls,
- the insurmountable barrier of a staircase that leads to a toileting difficulty.

Yet the contribution architectural design might positively make to the lives of people with dementia is not at all clear (Keen, 1989). While Marshall (1998) confidently asserts 'that the built environment can have a fundamental effect on a person with dementia design for people with dementia ... has not been subjected to the scrutiny of research in the same way as medication, for example', Kitwood *et al* (1995), in a report on dementia and residential care, observed that the 'physical environment had little relationship with well-being'.

Despite a growth of interest in design, much of what is accepted as established thinking is little more than assumption. For example, Netten (1989) attempted to relate interior design to the ability of disoriented residents to find their way around. Her conclusion was that 'the issue does not appear clear cut'. Even the use of prosthetic orientation cues is of uncertain benefit. Woods (1996) notes that the use of colour, architectural and other features to distinguish areas within a unit has not been adequately evaluated. While those with early dementia may respond to and benefit from directional information, as dementia progresses signs, symbols and pathfinder cues are increasingly ignored to the point where some people may perceive them as unwelcome environmental 'noise' (clutter) and attempt to remove them.

The Contribution of Building Design

Despite the paucity of research, the basic position of all workers is that the buildings in some way influence the behaviour of people who live within them, even though opinion remains largely intuitive. Lawton & Simon (1968) put forward the 'environmental docility' hypothesis. In other words, the more incompetent and vulnerable a person is, the more their behaviour is controlled by the environment that surrounds them.

The implications of this line of argument for those with dementia are clear. They are among the least competent people. If they find themselves in unsupportive surroundings, a marked proportion of their dependent and dysfunctional behaviour can be attributed to their environment. Many years ago, Lindsley (1964) proposed the prosthetic environment, wherein skills and abilities which are damaged or lost are compensated for by the provision of environmental prostheses. 'If behaviour is deficient, the environment could be altered in order to produce effective behaviour.' In similar vein, the potential value of the 'empathic model' of design has been explored by Pastalan (1984). The model's general principles attempt to create living arrangements that are enabling, rather than disabling:

1   'Organised space as stimulus'. If recognition, recall or understanding have deteriorated make a design message available through more than one sensory modality. An example is a dining room where the clatter of knives and forks, smelling food and seeing crockery, dining tables and chairs all declare: 'This is where you eat!'
2   'Organised spaces as orientation'. Any space should have a singular and unambiguous use, for people with dementia are less able to resolve ambiguities.

The following case study describes how a creative intervention that employed the principles of the 'empathic model' of design resolved the violent reactions of a woman with severe dementia.

Case study: The sadness of Mrs O

Mrs O, aged 75 years and suffering from probable Alzheimer's disease, found intimate care distressing. Efforts to assist her in the toilet, attempting to change her wet clothing and dressing her leg ulcers were met with unbridled ferocity. Unbeknown to staff, Mrs O had been an abused child.

Prior to Mrs O's entering residential care, the district nurse dressed her legs, and on occasions she had taken her to the toilet. Not only was there no record of distressed behaviour, the notes documented how 'chatty' and 'jolly' she seemed. Now in care, in no way could it be said that she was anything other than traumatised by the experience of personal care. Why was it so different now she was in a residential home?

The medical model offered a solution: dementia is progressive. She was now more demented than before, and thus more disoriented, disinhibited and, in general, more difficult. Yet this was not the explanation.

What was perplexing was that Mrs O was reacting to a care regime that appeared both sensitive and, when taken at face value, appropriate to her needs. Care followed principles of home life. Staff rarely wore uniforms. During intimate care, her carers always promoted dignity and self-respect. For example, dressings would always be changed in the privacy of her bedroom; toilet doors would always be closed. These actions were to be admired, yet what were the implications for Mrs O, a woman with an abusive legacy? When her dressings needed to be changed she would be taken by a care worker, in her eyes a relative stranger, to the privacy of her room, sat on or by her bed, her skirt would be lifted and her stockings removed. In this setting, is it surprising that she feared what might happen next? Having lost reasoning and judgement, unable to recall, probably even understand the reassuring words of staff, Mrs O was incapable of appreciating the true nature of the experience. The abuse was no longer consigned to the experiences of many years ago. The passage of time could no longer temper her trauma, for there had been none. Ribot's law had seen to that. The psychological context was both painful and 'now'. To be toileted was equally distressing, for again she was confronted by somebody attempting to 'remove' her clothes.

Drawing upon the 'empathic model', it was decided to 'medicalise' her care. Mrs O had accepted the home visits from the district nurse, not because she was less demented, but because she was less threatened. The nurse turned up in her uniform. There was little chance of misinterpretation. Armed with this understanding, from now on, when her dressings needed to be changed, Mrs O was not taken to her room but guided instead to the rarely used 'treatment room'. When she was sitting next to the medical trolley, cued into the clinical experience by an excess of bandages, dressings and the smell of ointments, the potential for misunderstanding was reduced. The space had an unambiguous, non-threatening use: no trauma, no anger; instead, peace of mind was observed.

Learning from these lessons, the staff took advantage of the treatment room's anxiety-reducing cues to address Mrs O's toileting difficulty. A programme of three-hourly visits to the toilet was implemented. This fixed schedule required Mrs O to be taken however, not to the toilet, but to the treatment room. While sitting next to the dressings trolley, her keyworker would talk to her. Not that the content of the conversation was important; Mrs O was soothed by the reassuring use of body language, facial expression and voice tone. When calm, she would be taken across the room to where a commode had been placed behind a screen. Reassured by the abundant cues of the treatment room, Mrs O's behaviour bore testimony to how safe she felt: no violence, just benign acceptance.

This use of the empathic model demonstrates that there are few, if any set ways of working with those who have dementia, just guidelines and intuition. In this instance person-centred resolution followed the introduction of a programme of care that was reminiscent of past institutional practice. Yet for Mrs O, her need for security was met. (For a more detailed account of Mrs O's history see Stokes, 1997.)

Other design features that contribute towards quality care, and which by their absence, may either cause or contribute to the onset of challenging behaviour are considered below.

The intimacy gradient In a residential or nursing home people need a gradient of settings which have different degrees of intimacy. A bedroom is most intimate; a lounge in a group-living unit less so; a communal sitting-room more public still; the front entrance area most public of all. All buildings which accommodate people need a definite gradient from 'front' to 'back', from the most public spaces at the front to the most intimate areas at the rear.

The layout of space within a building should create a sequence which begins with the entrance and the most public parts of the building, then leads into more private areas and finally to the most private domains. Each person should have a room of their own where they can retire to be alone among treasured possessions, where they can be in receipt of personal care (never forgetting that person-centred principles only allow for practice guidelines, not prescribed approaches, as evidenced by the case of Mrs O) and which allows families to be intimate with their loved one. This need is fundamental and essential and a natural complement to the social world of continuing care. 'A room of one's own' (Alexander *et al,* 1977) should be located at the end of the intimacy gradient, far from communal areas. Such a living arrangement encourages staff to regard people with dementia as valued individuals with a right to privacy and respect. Toilets should be placed between day activity areas and private realms, so that both residents themselves and care staff assisting those who are highly dependent can reach them with ease and with minimal social attention.

Without a gradient of intimacy, care actions are often inappropriate to context. Intimate behaviours such as toileting may take place next to a front entrance, while access to a sleeping area may be open to visitors and staff on arrival. Shared bedrooms result in people waking up with a stranger in their midst. Such a poor fit between a person and their environment can result in distressed, defensive and unco-operative behaviours, for the subjective experience is both perplexing and intimidating.

Corridors The time a resident spends between rooms can be as important as the moments spent within rooms. A corridor which is long, devoid of natural light and bare of furnishings is consistent with our worst ideas of what is meant by 'institution'. A corridor may be considered too long when it is more than 50 feet in length. Spivack (1967) described how long corridors distort the perception of distance, interfere with verbal communication, obscure perception of the human figure and face, and generate anxiety and fear as a result of feeling enclosed. The potential for disorientation, conflict and unsafe interaction is described by Pennington (1996). To design out these effects, corridors should be kept short, benefit from natural light and be areas of interest. Corridors should be made as much like rooms as possible, with carpets, furniture, book shelves and small tables, and where sections of walls have been stepped out create places to lean and even sit. Themed corridors 'full of things to look at and touch' (Bignall, 1996) encourage people to linger with purpose, possibly even with a sense of fun. As a result, they cease to be experienced as passages and become very much a part of the living space of the building, supporting the rhythm of daily life.

Interior design Condemning people with dementia to live in anonymous, sterile surroundings compounds their inability to transform the unfamiliar to the familiar, and hence ensures the strangeness of their existence. While orientation cues may only benefit the minority, there is nothing to be lost, and possibly something to be gained by building directional prosthetics into interior design. If just one person is spared the indignity of roaming around wet and soiled, such intervention is to be valued.

Wall coverings and carpets can be used to distinguish zones within a continuing care setting, as can the use of soothing background music or aromas. Irving (1996) reports the benefits of wooden hand-rails that have been grooved to identify different areas, while Handysides (1993) describes a nursing home where the floors in different parts of the building feel and sound different.

To compensate for the loss of ability to understand the meaning of the written word, doors to rooms that are fundamental to daily life (for example, toilets) may be distinguished by colour coding or through the use of unique handle designs (for example, shape and texture).

Placing either photographs of the resident or their family, possibly from years gone by, or pictures relevant to their significant interests or milestone experiences, may serve to individualise bedroom doors.

Space There is a need for ample safe space for walking indoors and outdoors. When the boundaries of the building are reached, a sense of arrival rather than containment should be experienced (Harding & Jolley, 1994). Panoramic windows that open up views and encourage movement between the inside and enclosed walking areas outside contribute to a sense of freedom. Yet space should not be seen as simply enabling people to move around freely, it should also provide areas of sanctuary and quiet, where people can escape from the challenging behaviour of others. A building should also make available oases of interest, and nooks and crannies which encourage people to sit and linger. Every corner of a building is a potential sitting space, but each sitting space has different needs for comfort and enclosure according to its position in the 'intimacy gradient' (Alexander *et al*, 1977). Hence we move away from the tendency to think solely about *rooms* where people sit, and acknowledge that human activity naturally occurs throughout the building at a variety of degrees of intensity and intimacy.

An understandable reaction to the traditional design of institutions so long associated with poor quality care, with their echoing, featureless corridors, uniform colour schemes, high ceilings, communal living areas and lack of private space, has been the development of small, domestic special care units for people with dementia (Handysides, 1993; Woods, 1996). While they represent a major improvement in the built environment, and there is much in the various group-living designs to admire, in the realm of challenging behaviour the pendulum may have swung too far. Life within a small lounge may easily trigger aggressive confrontations. In the absence of walking paths there is a pervasive sense of confinement characterised by agitated pacing or forlorn hovering around doors waiting to 'escape'. Behaviour that is tolerated when there is space to get away and find sanctuary can be interpreted as unacceptable when confined within the boundary of a small unit. For example, Mr T would shout and scream throughout the day to a point where he would be abused by other residents. His conduct drove nursing staff to despair. While we were unable to unearth the probable explanation, although it was possibly related to self-stimulation when alone and communication when engaged (an impossible situation to resolve), his behaviour had not deteriorated since his arrival at the home. Mr T had behaved in this way for nearly 18 months, yet when he was living in the asylum on a large Nightingale ward, his behaviour was less invasive and thus more easily ignored. In his new surroundings his behaviour was redefined as unacceptably disruptive – a clear example of the way behaviour interpreted as challenging cannot be divorced from the perceptions of others.

Decision points Whilst space for people to use and staff to exploit creatively contributes to the well-being of residents, we cannot ignore the observation that distance and complexity contribute to problems of disorientation, wandering and toileting difficulty. Environments should help facilitate any improvement possible and slow down the rate of deterioration. An important feature enabling this goal is the degree of control a person has over their life, manifested in their capacity to navigate their way around the 'functional environment' of bedrooms, sitting areas, dining rooms and toilets (Netten, 1989). The functional routes within homes consist of pathways linking these areas, all of which are likely to present the person with choice points whenever there is a junction of corridors. Similarly, decisions will have to be made when a person is faced with exits from these areas.

Netten (ibid) found, unsurprisingly, that the more light there is, the more able a resident will be to find their way around. Meaningful landmarks also aid orientation. Unhelpful designs are those involving a lot of 'meaningless decisions', such as when there are long corridors with lots of doors, or when several short corridors form a 'maze' effect.

Visual access This is 'The capacity of residents to see or sense where they are – or want to go' (Judd, 1998). With damaged memory, those with dementia cannot remember what is around the corner, through that door, or even where they came from. As they walk, or are accompanied around the building, agitated, disoriented, even resistive, behaviour may occur. Clear visual paths may calm behaviour. To see your destination brings reassurance, helps maintain purpose and compensates for the fragmentation of experience. As Judd (ibid) notes, visual access is a close design ally of cues, making the environment 'legible'.

When a building is compatible with the needs of those who live within the architecture, then life quality can be further enhanced through micro-initiatives.

Flooring People with dementia prefer, as we do, carpets. They are warm, soft, homely and absorb extraneous noise (Harding, 1995).

Curtains Hanging bedroom curtains made of thick material blocks out street light, prevents shadows that can be misinterpreted and encourages sleep.

Lighting Glare and shadows disorientate; strip lights are synonymous with institutional care. Soft tone lighting generates a sense of warmth, while an illuminated fish tank provides gentle, diffuse light. Harding (ibid) suggests that strip lights can be concealed in false ceilings, providing the opportunity for illuminated colour in design. At night, low intensity lights on the landing, or in the corridors or hall, reduce disorientation and agitation, as well as helping to prevent accidents.

Colour Poor visual acuity means that strong contrasts of pattern and colour should be avoided. They can be perplexing and, when used in flooring, can be perceived as a step or a gap to be negotiated, thereby inhibiting movement.

Seating arrangements Breaking up space into small social areas through the creation of sitting circles can double the level of social contact (Stokes, 1990b). This contrasts with the sterile waiting room design which results in silent and withdrawn residents. Nothing ever happens, aside from the unexpected outbreak of calling out and apparently aimless walking around.

To anchor this seating arrangement there needs to be a natural focus. A television can be inappropriate as it may be an unwelcome source of environmental 'noise' and misinterpretation. There is no substitute for an artificial fire which appears alive and flickering within a room. Fire can be an emotional touchstone generating feelings of homeliness and comfort. Acting as a magnet, a fire attracts people to a room and makes it more likely for people to gather.

Eating atmosphere The inhospitable institutional feel of a dining room can be transformed through the provision of soft light, hung low over a table. When 'this one point of light lights up people's faces ... then a meal can become a special thing indeed, a bond, communion' (Alexander *et al*, 1977). It invites people to relax, and eat leisurely, rather than forcing them to eat in an atmosphere of noise and functional haste, feeling ill at ease, with a desire to walk away.

Harding & Jolley (1994) describe the piloting of design guidelines which would further contribute to the special needs and quality of life of those with dementia.

The Building: An Obstacle or Opportunity?

It is naïve to propose a deterministic view of the relationship between buildings and people who live in them. Such crude architectural determinism is flawed for buildings and designs are only as important as the manner in which they may or may not be used and the constraints and opportunities they present. Buildings can hinder or help the provision of quality care; in extreme cases they can prevent it, but, to state the obvious, buildings by themselves cannot provide it (Pennington, 1996). Arie (1987) asserts that, 'given a basic adequacy of material environment' quality of care depends on staff morale, motivation and training. Hence it can be confidently argued that the quality of the interpersonal environment is of greater importance than the physical, for negative staff attitudes will negate the effects of even the best architectural design (Woods, 1996).

The *domus* philosophy of residential care for elderly people with dementia was developed by Elaine Murphy and Alastair McDonald in the Lewisham and North Southwark Health District, London towards the end of the 1980s. While statements were made about building design and unit size, an early domus was housed in a modern three-storey hospital building, yet the domus philosophy of care (see Box 5.1) prevailed, with demonstrable benefit for residents (Lindesay *et al*, 1991). This is not altogether surprising, for it is not even clear whether 'home', an emotional touchstone inextricably related to security, sanctuary and a place to be ourselves, has any value in discussions of the physical characteristics of buildings (Keen, 1989). We know little about the detail of what people with dementia require of a building design to make it feel like home. What can be said is that there is undoubtedly a distinction between a 'homely' environment which is reflected in size and interior layout, and 'home' which is less to do with décor and decoration, and more to do with interpersonal relations and psychological attachments. Thus, while we can be enthusiastic (or unenthusiastic) about a building, quality of life is dependent upon the ability and desire of staff to construct sensitive and meaningful relationships with those in their care.

The warehousing of people with dementia can occur regardless of design, for institutionalisation is as much, if not more the consequence of staff attitudes and actions, as it is the result of architecture. While certain built environments may encourage positive caring behaviours (see, for example, Fallowfield, 1990), no design will ensure these will happen.

Box 5.1 The domus philosophy
- The domus is the resident's home for life.
- The needs of the staff are as important as those of the residents.
- The domus should aim to correct the avoidable consequences of dementia, and accommodate those that are unavoidable.
- The residents' individual psychological and emotional needs may take precedence over the physical aspects of their care.

The Social Environment

There is clear convergence between the various accounts that address the positive characteristics of caregiving (see Box 5.2), yet the poor quality of life for elderly people with dementia in permanent care has been demonstrated time and time again. Devaluation, invalidation and dehumanisation have often been described (Woods, 1995). Townsend (1962) identified six different aspects of institutional life:

- loss of activity and purpose
- isolation from family, friends and community
- tenuous relationships
- loneliness
- loss of privacy and identity
- collapse of self-determination.

Nearly 40 years on, these remain relevant issues. Why? Lindesay *et al* (1991) make reference to a process of 'institutional maintenance' whereby procedures and routines benefit the smooth running of the institution rather than the needs of those who live in them. We see a preoccupation with safety, hygiene and administration. As a consequence, residents' freedoms are limited, and carer's time is taken up with basic

---

Box 5.2 Positive characteristics of care

1 To respect and respond to individual need.

2 To promote life quality through the provision of personal control and choice.

3 To provide opportunity for independent behaviour and age-appropriate activity that is relevant and rewarding to the individual.

4 To maintain dignity.
(Stokes, 1990b)

1 Observing the early manifestations of ill-being.

2 Being able to intervene when interaction turns into confrontation.

3 Being there when walking turns into tottering.

4 Promoting independence.

5 Fostering well-being.

6 Encouraging competence.

7 Nurturing a therapeutic social environment.
(Pennington, 1996)

Care is concerned primarily with the maintenance and enhancement of personhood. Providing a safe environment, meeting basic needs and giving physical care are all essential, but only part of the care of the whole person. (Kitwood, 1995)

1 It values the person with dementia as a full human being.

2 The individualization of care requires getting to know the whole person.

3 Achieve effective two-way communication. (Woods, 1995)

---

physical and domestic tasks, while managerial time is devoted to service bureaucracy. Negative staff attitudes towards 'dementia' dominate. As a result, depersonalising practices and routines characterise daily life, there is a failure to recognise or meet individual need, and a culture of management, containment and control prevails. Contact between carers and the person with dementia is inevitably functional and perfunctory.

Kitwood (1990) refers to the 'processes and interactions that tend to depersonalize a sufferer from dementia' as the 'malignant social psychology', a significant non-biological influence on dementia, that is founded on the biomedical framework of a person suffering from a brain disease for which nothing can be done. Therapeutic nihilism dominates as carers believe such residents do not experience life or suffering and solely require basic physical care; there is no point trying to achieve anything more positive. Koch & Webb (1996) refer to 'conveyor belt care' that objectifies the person, adopts 'inflexible routines and offers privation of care other than basic physical interventions'. A culture of care that is ignorant and heartless, condemning many to a futile and loveless existence (Kitwood *et al*, 1995).

The Malignant Social Psychology

In 1990, Kitwood proposed these two fundamental equations

$$SD = NI + MSP$$

(senile dementia is compounded from the effects of neurological impairment and of malignant social psychology)

$$(NI)_a \leftarrow MSP$$

(neurological impairment in an elderly person attracts to itself a malignant psychology)

In so doing he articulated what was intuitively known, namely that, when 'we follow any person's dementing illness carefully, observing its course in the realities of everyday life, it is extremely difficult to conclude that we are simply witnessing the inexorable consequences of a process of degeneration in nervous tissue' (Kitwood, 1996). Although in other writings, Kitwood (1993) acknowledged a complex interaction between five factors that had been previously elucidated by Stokes & Allen (1990):

$$\text{Senile Dementia} = \text{Personality (P)} + \text{Biography (B)} + \text{Health (H)}$$
$$+ \text{Neurological Impairment (NI)}$$
$$+ \text{Social Psychology (SP)}$$

it is Kitwood's contention that the progression of dementia depends primarily on the interplay between neurological impairment and social psychology – a social psychology interpreted, not as an academic discipline, but as an entity (Morton, 1997).

A person with dementia lives within a human context, exposed to interpersonal interactions and relationships. Those who are being cared for by a spouse or family are in receipt of tenderness and love founded on deeply rooted relationships. Yet their way of being may challenge the limits of others' endurance and understanding. Pre-existing family tensions may be intensified. Those in 'formal' care are liable to some degree of 'institutional maintenance' while experiencing a social world that is little more than a collectivity of strangers, some of whom will be truly strange.

While Kitwood's concept of a malignant social psychology is most applicable to the inadequacy of care (see Box 5.3), it needs to be acknowledged that malignancy is to be found in the social grouping of dementia. In other words, anyone who has dementia may be distressed or devalued by the actions of those who care for them, as well as those alongside whom they live, as well as by those who care for them.

Episodes detailed in Box 5.3 or observed, for example in the case of Patrick (p51) are not specific to care within institutions, but may characterise the nature of any caregiving relationship. Tragically, for the consequences may be devastating, 'the malignant social psychology is so much a part of the taken-for-granted world of later life that it generally passes unnoticed' (Kitwood, 1990). For, while the actions may be commonplace, a malignant social psychology is seldom the result of malicious intent.

Kitwood (ibid) addresses why dementia should attract to itself a malignant social psychology and identifies four related reasons:

1   Absence of empathy for the person with dementia.
2   The pressure and burden of responsibility and unremitting demands that generates, especially among family caregivers, a sense of living a 36-hour day (Mace & Rabins, 1992). Short staffing in continuing care contributes to the staff's sense of exhaustion.
3   As those with dementia appear so different from their previous selves, 'there is a tendency not to believe in the sufferer from dementia as a person, and so not to treat him or her with the respect that properly accords to persons'. When one holds the belief that dementia leaves behind a 'shell' of a person, then 'how I relate to this "person" matters little'.
4   A defence against the fear and anxiety that disability might arouse. By detaching oneself from the reality of dementia, in other words invoking the social distance, a caregiver can say, 'I will never be like that.'

This framework for dementia has similarities to social models of disability wherein the attitudes of people towards a person perceived as different actively disempower the person with disability and deny them a voice, thus exacerbating existing disabilities and attracting even more negative attitudes.

Box 5.3 Kitwood's malignant social psychology

Aspect	Description
Accusation	The person is blamed for action, or failure to act, which result from their loss of skills or inability to understand the situation.
Banishment	The person is either sent away or excluded – either physically, psychologically, or both – thus depriving them of sustaining human contact.
Disempowerment	The person is not allowed to utilise their remaining abilities. They do not receive assistance to complete actions they have initiated.
Disparagement	The person is given messages that they are incompetent, a failure and so on. This damages their self-esteem.
Disruption	The person experiences a sudden disturbance to their frame of reference while in the middle of an action or reflection.
Ignoring	Carrying on conversation or actions as if the person were not present.
Imposition	Overriding the desires of, or denying choice to, a person.
Infantilisation	Treating a person very patronisingly, as if they were a young child.
Intimidation	A person is made fearful by threats, physical power or by being placed in situations in which they are unable to make sense of their surroundings.

Invalidation	The person's subjectivity, especially their feelings, is either denied, not acknowledged or dismissed as insignificant.
Labelling	The diagnostic category becomes the foundation for attempts to understand, and attempts to communicate with, a person.
Mockery	A person's disabilities are used as a source of humour.
Objectification	A person's status as a sentient human being is disregarded. They are treated as if they are not really present.
Outpacing	A person is excluded by those around them acting and speaking at a pace which leaves them bewildered.
Stigmatisation	The person is treated as an outcast.
Treachery	Trickery and deception are used in order to manipulate a person into behaving in a way that is desired by others.
Withholding	A person's physical and psychological needs are disregarded.

Kitwood (1990) even considers that the malignant social psychology may play a causal role in bringing about neurological impairment, inasmuch as psychological aspects of the environment may well be as 'dementogenic' as physical factors. How structural changes within the brain can be brought about by continual and disastrous psychological damage remains an area of contentious debate, yet this radical proposal need not detract from the central argument that the quality of care has a significant impact, for better or worse, on the process of dementia.

For Kitwood, a profound consequence of the malignant social psychology is the loss of personhood. For personhood to be maintained 'an individual needs not only to be in relationship [with others] but also to be accorded status ... In terms of social status, it requires an acknowledgement of one's subjectivity and uniqueness as an individual' (Kitwood, 1994). An individual needs to be 'treated like a real person with their feelings acknowledged and their point of view valued' (Morton,

1999). The denial of personhood, on the other hand, is experienced when others do not acknowledge your presence and act as if you are unworthy of respect. The malignant social psychology is 'inimical to replenishment of personhood' (ibid). While a cognitively intact person can attempt to remedy or avoid such malignancy, and seek replenishment of their personhood elsewhere, 'the person with lowered competence and function is more likely to be shaped by and vulnerable to 'environmental influences' (Woods, 1996). At the mercy of their social surroundings, 'there is a dismantling of personality, a loss of self' (Kitwood, 1990).

Abuse, Maltreatment and Insensitivity: a Continuum of Malignancy

Much has been said about the insensitive and dehumanising 'taken-for-granted world of care', driven by good intentions, yet unwittingly corrosive, a malignant social environment eloquently described by Tom Kitwood and his colleagues at the Bradford Dementia Group. Yet not all care that is destructive and damaging is without malevolent intent. While levels of elder abuse (for example, neglect, physical assault, sexual abuse and financial exploitation) are thankfully low, or at least the reporting of episodes is uncommon, abuse of older adults is 'acknowledged as a social problem in need of remediation' (Kingston & Reay, 1996). Accepting that there are difficulties of definition and reporting inaccuracies, Ogg & Bennett (1992) found that two per cent of older people living at home in the United Kingdom had been physically abused, while a US study established that 40 per cent of staff working in residential homes admitted committing acts of psychological abuse, and 10 per cent acknowledged actions of physical abuse (Pillemer & Moore, 1989). More alarmingly, Cooney & Howard (1995) suggest that 'Elderly people with dementia living with a carer are at a significantly higher risk of abuse than the general population over 65'. One study reported that nearly 12 per cent of carers had physically abused their relative (Coyne *et al*, 1993).

Between the extremes of obvious abuse and the taken for granted world of malign care (Box 5.3) there lies maltreatment, deliberate, knowing actions that are damaging to those who are vulnerable. What distinguishes these from abusive acts is that abuse, when exposed, is condemned, while maltreatment is condoned and accepted. To the enlightened the case examples that follow resonate with a sense of abuse, not impoverished care. Yet these actions were known, tolerated and advocated by the involved caregivers, sometimes for years.

Case Study 1

A relief homecare worker had just completed her tasks of caring. The elderly woman had been dressed, washed and been assisted to the toilet. Having helped her husband prepare breakfast for them both, the carer was about to leave when the man reminded her to 'use the elastic'. When she looked bemused, the husband handed her an elasticated cord which, he explained would be needed to confine his wife to her chair. When she refused, he demanded that she do as he asked, otherwise he would not be able to get on with his life: she followed him around; if he went out she would be in the street searching; he could not leave her alone in the house, there was the cooker, the taps, the fire ... The homecare worker telephoned her manager who confirmed this was an appropriate course of action and had been so for nearly 18 months: it was what the husband needed, and at least his wife would be safe. The homecare worker contacted the Inspection Unit.

Case Study 2

A 'bathing batch' was seen as an effective and efficient way to bathe six residents in less than 30 minutes, using just two members of staff. Picture the scene. In the bathroom there are three naked residents. One is being removed from the bath, while another is being helped in. The water has not been changed. Sitting on a chair is a resident who will be the next one to be bathed.

As the resident who was first out of the bath leaves the room, she will pass three residents sitting on chairs with towels around them, one of whom will replace her in the bathroom. Within a short while all will have been 'bathed'. On only a few occasions will the bath have been topped up with warm water. The bath will never have been emptied and refilled.

This practice was in effect for over five years in a residential home for the care of 'the elderly mentally infirm'.

Case Study 3

It is around 7.30pm and it is time for the 12 residents of the dementia care unit to retire for the night. They are roused from their slumbers and directed towards the bedroom area. The built design is small-scale, homely in style, with single rooms big enough for plenty of personal possessions. Much corresponds to good design for dementia (Marshall, 1998). As they walk along the corridor, the disoriented and dependent residents come across four commodes positioned against the walls, in pairs facing each other. The first four residents are placed on the commodes, while the rest are held back. When, and only when, there is evidence of urination and/or defecation is the person removed and they continue their journey to their bedroom. Those who are waiting will now replace those who have 'passed through' the commodes. This is seen as an effective way of ensuring that all residents are toileted before bed, thereby minimising night-time bed wetting and nocturnal disturbance.

This procedure was not hidden from managers. It was known and considered to be an appropriate way of caring for people with dementia: are they not oblivious to their surroundings and unresponsive to what goes on around them? Is it not best to ensure their physical welfare and save them the discomfort of lying in a soiled bed?

As can be seen from the above examples, the difference between abuse and maltreatment is clear. The former is condemned and the perpetrators are held to account, the latter is condoned and the practice accepted. Yet what is the emotional experience of such degrading care? What reactions should we expect?

Well-Being in Dementia

We do not need to be told when the quality of dementia care is poor, where people are treated en bloc, as if they have the same needs; where little effort is made to preserve dignity; where they are 'treated as a passive, inanimate object to be cleaned and changed in a dehumanizing manner' (Woods, 1996), for those with dementia are superb barometers of the quality of care. Kitwood (1995) describes the 'sense of deadness, apathy, boredom, gloom and fear; most of those being cared for appear to have given up hope, their last resort being an occasional moan, or shout, or angry outburst'.

Where negative emotion dominates we talk of a state of ill-being (Buckland, 1997), a state characterised by restless agitation, screaming, anger and overt hostility. When a person's life is dominated by regimented patterns of care or they are exposed to a social world characterised by a loss of regard for the person, such 'acting-out behaviours' are easy to understand. Kitwood *et al* (1995) found higher levels of ill-being where there was an emphasis on staff routines and procedures. However, what is often observed is a state of apparent indifference, not overt distress or hostility. Is it true then, that those with dementia are unaffected by their experience? Many people have commented how struck they are by the emotional indifference of those with dementia (for example, Gilleard, 1984), the interpretation being that they are untroubled by the experience, and that when insight is lost, the 'worst is behind them'. How wrong we have been. Their apparent indifference is consistent with what is known of victim responses. Victims of abuse, regardless of its nature, rarely, if ever, fight back. In the beginning there may have been resistance and protest, but eventually this is replaced by passive resignation. They are weak, the abuser is powerful. They no longer resist or recoil, but enter a world of semi-depressed withdrawal, seemingly indifferent to their fate.

It is to be hoped that people with dementia are not victims of abuse, yet they are victims of circumstances. They do not wish to be among those who, in their eyes, are not like them; to be confronted with depersonalised, disempowering care actions; to be deprived of personal respect. They do not wish to be alone in a mysterious world of not knowing. Whilst in the beginning, they may have protested – hitting out, shouting, trying to leave – they soon present as accepting and indifferent. Yet this cannot be interpreted as evidence of positive adjustment, to be defined as 'settling down'. We should be as concerned for those who are passive, silent and disengaged as we are for those who are demonstrably suffering. The *victim response* is in many ways the most common and demanding manifestation of challenging behaviour encountered in dementia care (see Moniz-Cook, 1998). Kitwood *et al* (1995) profile 'Eve', a woman who I believe characterises the typical profile of a victim:

She is easily upset and often very anxious. She does not make friends with other people, and does not like to do anything at all. Staff find

> that most people like Eve are very difficult to relate to, however Eve has a vulnerability about her … Most of the time Eve is withdrawn into herself, and closed to all around.

She has not settled. Yes, she is quiet, passive, but also demonstrably troubled. Nor can we automatically offer a biogenic explanation for her 'lack of behaviour'. The cerebral disease is not exacting an increasingly challenging toll on her capacity to function. Instead, we can acknowledge that her presentation reveals her suffering, not her emotional indifference.

A culture of care that frees itself from the shackles of the 'standard paradigm' and strives to maintain a state of relative well-being (Kitwood *et al*, 1995) is concerned with the quality of human relationships, a culture not founded on principles of control, containment and management, but on sensitivity, empathy and resolution. Kitwood (1995) contrasts the 'old' and 'new' cultures of care, observing that today we need to acknowledge that those who have dementia are equal members of the human race, for whom care should be concerned primarily with the maintenance and enhancement of personhood. The key elements of such 'positive person work' that make for well-being (see Kitwood, 1996) include providing a place that is safe and secure ('holding'); acceptance of the 'personal truth' of their experience ('validation'); enabling people to do what they otherwise might not be able to do ('facilitation'); engaging in meaningful, enjoyable human contact as distinct from adopting traditional 'parent-child' relationships ('celebration'); and the pleasurable stimulation of the senses ('stimulation').

Is it possible, however, to know when a state of relative well-being is attained? The answer is a cautious 'yes'. Buckland (1997) details those behaviours which intuitively would only likely occur if a person was feeling a state of well-being. These include assertiveness, initiating social contact, affection, sensitivity to others, self-respect, relaxation, helpfulness, creativity and humour: characteristics that are so often either absent or encountered at a 'trace level'.

However, when observed, are we working with fleeting phenomena? Is it the case that, when the gentle touch, the smile, the reassuring words are forgotten, the magic of the moment is lost? If so, then that does not in any way decry the efforts made to bring peace of mind and pleasure to those who are troubled. We work with the 'now', and if we can bring contentment and relative joy into the fragmented lives of those who are dementing for just a moment then that is to be valued. But possibly the answer is a tentative 'no'. Kitwood (1996) reports that when human relationships 'make for well-being, we have often observed that when this has consistently been in operation for, say, half an hour, a person gains enough confidence and security to cope well for the two or three hours that follow, as if personhood has temporarily been restored'.

So are our efforts to promote well-being more lasting than we might have thought? What can be said is this: a person sitting next to one who screams and lashes out for no reason will show signs of physiological arousal on whatever measure we choose for minutes after the upsetting event – long after the experience has been forgotten. In other words, distress persists beyond the survival of the memory trace. So why should the opposite not apply? Maybe we do not simply work in the immediacy of the moment, but in a world which, though transient and brief, is not as fleeting as we may imagine.

The delivery of person-centred care is not easy. It is demanding and requires a greater degree of empathy and identification with the person with dementia than is traditionally observed. That resident who is unco-operative, always resisting when we wish to take her to the toilet or to the dining table – is her behaviour that surprising? Does she deserve to be labelled as resistive? Would you willingly go with strangers, even if they smiled and tempted you with fine words? Behind the barrier of shattered memory and devastated understanding that is who we are: strangers with little to offer other than mysterious intent. We protest that they are people like ourselves, then expect them to do what we could never do – not simply to go with those they do not know, but often to receive intimate care when they are incapable of knowing their own deficiencies. We expect them to accept a level of personal hygiene different from our own, for why else do we have the reassuring availability of staff toilets? Yet dementing people do not have insight into their condition. They cannot make allowances when they are unaware of their failings. Is this why some avoid using the communal toilets (remember Mrs S, pp52–3). What is it like to be stopped from leaving a building when all around you is chaos and noise; or finding a person in your home who reassures you that you are safe but then requests you to sit down and not leave. Despite the role and title of homecare worker, to you she is a stranger. And what would you have done if, on waking this morning a person you had never seen before had told you to stay indoors? Might you have protested, attempted to 'escape', demanded to know their identity and insisted that they leave? You do not have to be dementing to act in such a way, but to do so when you are will result in others degrading your actions to the status of symptoms and labelling you as a 'changed person': aggressive, violent, abusive, noisy, a wanderer.

Then there is the night. Can we imagine lying in bed and hearing voices and footsteps outside the bedroom, or seeing a shaft of light seeping under the door? They do not know they are in care. What sense can they make of the situation? We have never gone to bed in such circumstances. We close down the house before retiring at night so it is dark, quiet and, most importantly, secure. Is it little wonder they are prompted to investigate? Are we witnessing nocturnal disturbance, or an understandable need to know and gain peace of mind? And then there is Joyce, whose distress demonstrates the challenge of person-centred work and the unfulfilled need for empathy.

All morning Joyce has been demanding to know where her husband has gone. In the beginning, staff were sensitive, gently communicating that Len had died five years earlier. She would walk away, silent yet clearly disbelieving. Within moments she would return, pleading to know his whereabouts, demanding to know why you will not search for him. Patience is stretched to the limit. Sensitivity and understanding fade. 'Joyce, we've told you a dozen times …'; 'How many more times must we tell you …'; 'Joyce, you know Len is dead …'. Now she no longer walks away, there is confrontation. At that point, the telephone in the office rings. You are nearest. It is the police. Tragically, on the way to work this morning the husband of one of your colleagues has been killed in a road traffic accident. The police are still at the scene of the accident, and will be for some time. They do not wish your colleague to find out accidentally that her husband is dead. Would you kindly inform her? You put down the telephone and with a degree of foreboding you cross the office floor. You have to break this terrible news to your colleague. As you enter the corridor, to your right, there she is, walking towards you. At the same moment, to your left, you see Joyce coming your way. You know what she wants; you know what she will ask: 'Where's my husband?' At this point, will you demonstrate as much sensitivity and compassion to Joyce as you are now going to show to your colleague? She is a person like ourselves. As Kitwood (1995) describes, an equal member of the human race, yet the answer is possibly not. As has been pointed out, person-centred care is easier to articulate than it is to deliver.

An Holistic Model of Explanation

The model of understanding is complete, an understanding that is far removed from the reductionist explanation provided by the 'standard

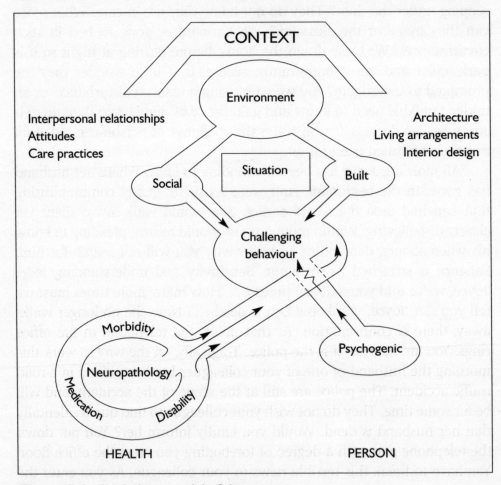

Figure 5.1 *The holistic model of dementia.*

paradigm'. Compare the medical model displayed in Figure 5.1. The explanatory pathways responsible for what we know as dementia are clear to see.

We have moved far away from a nihilistic disease model to the description of a framework that enables us to develop cultures of care that acknowledge the person and identify the potential for change. The pathways enable us to recognise that challenging behaviour is not of mysterious origin. Rather, it reveals the struggles of those who are attempting to live their lives in the face of neurological adversity in settings ill-equipped either to respect their personhood or to respond to their needs. No explanation of dementia can stand without reference to these roots. Neuropathology inaugurates the cognitive decline that the person, misunderstood and then denied, brings to a pitiless consummation. We forsake the negative parameters of the standard paradigm and strive to restore the person, thereby addressing the therapeutic potential of resolution.

CHAPTER 6
The Needs of People with Dementia

AS OUR UNDERSTANDING of challenging behaviour has progressed over the past decade or so, the language has correspondingly changed. The terms 'management' and 'problems', and reference to 'difficult', or 'anti-social' behaviour have been replaced by a concern for meaning and an acceptance that we are often working with a person whose needs are neither met nor acknowledged.

Kitwood (1995) highlights the point that, in the old culture of care, problem behaviours 'must be managed skilfully and efficiently'. This language of control reflected a desire to contain the consequences of unwanted, annoying behaviour, rather than seeking 'to understand the message, and so to engage with the need that is not being met'.

With the appreciation that challenging behaviour could not 'be attributed solely to organic changes within the brain' (Stokes, 1987a) and an understanding of the richness of potential explanation (Stokes, 1986a; 1986b; 1987a; 1987b), while the language of intervention was that of the 'management of problems', it gradually became evident that understanding was revealing a realm of human need that was denied by others. This resulted in inarticulate communication and forlorn efforts on the part of those with dementia to express these drives and desires (Goudie & Stokes, 1989; Stokes & Goudie, 1990). The message was clear: "know the person", otherwise the provision of care is unlikely to meet individual need' (Stokes

& Allen, 1990); 'Look behind what is said to uncover hidden meaning and feeling. Practise person-centred care' (Stokes, 1990d). Yet we needed to progress from understanding the reasons for challenging behaviour, but then doing no more than proceeding down the path of 'management'. Resolution had to be the objective.

The previous chapters have set the scene. A person with dementia has needs which are more typical of people in general than specific to those with dementia, needs that have been present since the formative times of our human development. Devoid of their mature correlates we may observe the purity of needs, distorted and disguised by cognitive decay, yet evidence of human qualities that may 'pertain to the "free child", who perhaps was hidden away for years behind layer and layer of repression' (Kitwood, 1996). If not hidden by repression, then by the effects of socialisation and conforming with age-appropriate expectations.

Physical Needs

We take it as given that all, regardless of their intellectual status require food, fluid, warmth and shelter. In the 'warehousing' culture so often observed, providing for these basic requirements is the benchmark of 'good care'. Yet even in this domain of need we may get it sadly wrong. Do we acknowledge residents' need to exercise – not to 'work out', but just to walk? Or are we too quick to see it as 'wandering'? Consider the need for personal hygiene and the plight of Mrs S (pp52–3). To what extent do you enjoy using public lavatories, or benefit from the availability of staff toilets? Your concern for cleanliness will not be eroded because of a failing memory. Yes, all people with dementia are one day rendered incontinent, but this is when we are considering the advance into total dependency. Prior to these times of degradation the motives to toilet will be strongly governed by values of cleanliness that we have carried with us since those early years when our parents impressed upon us the need to toilet hygienically and our aversion to communal toileting began.

Then there is the need to be free of pain. As described earlier (p63), this may result in a range of challenging behaviours, the origins of which may be sorely misunderstood. We work with those whose ability to communicate has been devastated by aphasia and dysarthria. They cannot effectively articulate their health needs, and yet dementia does not exercise miraculous protection from disease or disorder. It is well established that, as we age, the likelihood of ill-health and disability increases dramatically. So one would expect that assertive healthcare would characterise care regimes: well-person clinics would be held by family doctors or practice nurses, dentists, physiotherapists and chiropodists would regularly visit, not because there are identifiable problems, but to prevent ailments progressing in those who cannot report their discomfort and sensations. Yet we know this does not happen. People with dementia are the least likely to receive healthcare unless their condition becomes acute. And we are not necessarily talking about serious health problems. How well do we respond to the needs of those who suffer in 'silence' (or possibly not) from headache, toothache, earache, arthritis and so on? Ron had challenged our attempts to understand his tendency to be unpredictably violent. For three months we had searched for meaning and failed. One day, as an aside, a care assistant mentioned his broken and blackened teeth. I believe he had eight teeth extracted. Thereafter, he was never a saint, but his conduct dramatically improved. He had clearly been reacting to toothache. He needed a dentist, not thioridazine.

To neglect these fundamental physical needs is to provide compelling evidence that again we are examining practice that is not person-centred. Yes, we know something about them, but 'they are not truly like us'. If we confine people to chairs, 'ghettoise' their toileting arrangements and deny them appropriate healthcare, how can it be otherwise?

The Need for Security

This refers not so much to the perils of steep stairs, slippery floors and busy roads, as to the basic need for emotional security (for example, Erikson, 1963). The need to be psychologically safe is a powerful determinant of behaviour. This has been seen in the cases of Mr D (p64) and Mrs O (p78), and is also revealed in the case of Mrs D and the colour purple (see Box 6.1).

Box 6.1 Mrs D and the 'Colour Purple'

Client: Mrs D, aged 74 years.

Diagnosis: Probable Alzheimer's disease.

History: Has suffered from dementia for five years.

Circumstances:
Has lived in a social services EMI (elderly mentally infirm) unit for the past month, alongside nine people with dementia.

Presenting problem:
During the day Mrs D is pleasant and compliant. High dependency needs. At night, however, she will not stay in her bedroom. She persistently walks the corridor, enters the bedrooms of others or attempts to sleep in a chair in the lounge. Noisy, resistive and, on occasions, destructive if returned to her own room. Challenging behaviour present since admission.

Initial explanations:
1 Nocturnal disorientation.
2 Diurnal rhythm disturbance.
3 Attention seeking.

Action:
An increase in night-time sedation and the provision of a night light in her room.

Outcomes:
1 No reduction in disturbed behaviour at night, but more withdrawn during the day.
2 Mrs D is labelled as a 'wanderer' and 'aggressive'.

Revised formulation:
Mrs D is Irish and was once a devout Roman Catholic. The colour scheme of her bedroom is purple and mauve; in her faith these are the colours of mourning. Mrs D had always had a morbid dread of these colours and their distressing association with grief and death. Away from her bedroom, she was psychologically comfortable. However, when confronted with her room she was consumed by fear and insecurity, and sought sanctuary elsewhere.

Yet how safe can those with dementia feel in a world increasingly devoid of familiarity and reassurance, not simply because the novel will always remain so, but because Ribot's law destroys the last vestige of familiarity that remains? The answer is that most do not feel safe. Instead, we see separation anxiety, a negative emotion when apart from those people or that place that make us feel safe and secure. It is observed among children on their first day at nursery or school, or when we feel homesick. For people with dementia such feelings of separation characterise everyday life, even when objectively there is much around to provide security. Not, however in their subjective world of not knowing. The outcome may be a terror of being alone, agitated attempts to leave, demands to go home or plaintive cries for parents (see p66).

Insecurity arises not only from a subjective state of separation, but also because the world of dementia may in itself be truly fearful. Night is especially traumatic. Every waking moment is a time of not knowing, a time to face mysterious shadows and unexpected, inexplicable noises with no recall of where they are to comfort them. The darkness and solitude bring no hope of reassurance. It is little wonder we face the challenge of 'nocturnal disturbance'. Yet how does our irritation and exasperation compare with their panic and bewilderment?

Kitwood *et al* (1995) discuss how it is important 'to provide more stability, more of a sense of a continuing rhythm in daily life, if a person with dementia is to feel secure'. Devoid of 'inner stabilisation', a person can easily become disoriented and frightened. We can cope with discontinuity, and change that is sudden and unexpected, they cannot. Do we rise to the challenge and provide consistent care practice, the benefits of which are not so much that they get to know us and our ways, as that we get to know them? As we approach the person *we* know, we establish eye contact and smile. Their welcoming response can make us believe they know us well, when it is more than likely that they are responding to our interpersonal warmth. This is what Kitwood (1996) has referred to as 'holding'.

Studies of the growth of sociability (Schaffer, 1971) demonstrate that fear of the strange is not produced by social stimuli that are totally unfamiliar, but by experiences that combine the familiar and unfamiliar. People with dementia correspond to such stimuli, recognisable, yet strange at the same time – people whose outward appearance is acknowledged as familiar, but whose behaviour does not correspond to the cultural norms that govern social engagement, norms that are acquired in childhood experience, not by formal education, and hence will not be lost early in dementia.

Sitting in a communal lounge can we imagine what it might be like being next to a person who smears you with faeces or calls out for no reason? Or to be faced with a person who attempts to pull you out of your chair while calling you a name that is not yours or reaches over and takes food off your plate? Or to observe others lying on the floor, plucking at imaginary objects, or banging on windows or exposing themselves? To be exposed to these social experiences and possess no explanation as to what is happening or why you are in the midst of such bedlam?

Such fear and frustration will be increasingly met with immature and unsuccessful methods of solution. In maturity, cortical development and the concomitant exposure to learning and experience result in emotional behaviour that is integrated and controlled. In dementia, the cortical component in emotional responsiveness is progressively lost. As a result, the accompanying emotional reactions may be misunderstood by others in terms of their expression and ferocity, emotions that are essentially inborn and develop without any special opportunities for learning. The feelings register is broad and, when expressed, can be gross, immediate and unrestrained.

The feeling tone that accompanies the frustration of need may result in unbridled anger or destructive impulses, an excess of restless movement, apathy and withdrawal, agitated and repetitive actions, or regression to primitive and infantile actions, behaviour that is experienced as disproportionate, inexplicable, unacceptable, yet conduct typical of responses observed in dementia.

For those who adhere to the medical model a perverse error of judgement may now occur. When caring for a person with dementia on an in-patient assessment unit, or during a period of respite stay, or at a day centre, if these behaviours are interpreted as symptoms of dementia rather than being taken as demonstrable evidence that the person cannot cope in the company of those with dementia, these signs may be taken as the basis for declaring that 'we have discovered the true extent of their dementia', judging that care at home is no longer feasible, and then condemning them to *live with* those who have dementia!

Yet could it be that we are culpable in exacerbating their insecurity? Do we provide an interpersonal environment that is safe and secure? Do we truly 'hold' them? Even though our intentions are to be respected, on many occasions I think the answer is that we do not. Imagine the scene. A new client is being welcomed to a day centre, all around strange behaviour abounds. Yet is anything said to comfort or reassure? As the person is being told how they are going to enjoy themselves at the centre, how there are friends to make and much to do, and, significantly, that there is nothing to worry about, what is going on before them? Maybe there is somebody lying on the floor, another person crying out; two people are cursing each other and someone is removing their clothes. Nothing to worry about? It does not *feel* that way. Understandably, I think, their need is to leave. Is this unreasonable? Why do we cast a veil over the reality of the situation, ignore it as if it is not happening and instead indulge in platitudes?

The person with dementia is experiencing and feeling the situation accurately. Their actions are appropriate. It is we who are practising denial. It is we who are failing to construct bonds of trust, regardless of how tenuous these may be. Is this providing a psychologically safe environment within which a person can feel moments of security? Why are we not honest and open, informing them that, yes, it is happening, it is troubling, yet they are, all the same, safe; and then continuously replenishing their need to be secure? Would we not wish to be informed, to know that others are sharing the same experiences? Or would we wish to be abandoned in a mysterious world, that becomes even more frightening as our experiences remain unacknowledged?

The Need for Occupation

From the earliest days of life we need and benefit from stimulation. What do many parents put above the cot when they bring their new-born home from the maternity hospital? A mobile. It is colourful, it moves, it makes noises. To be engaged in occupation, whether it be passive or active, is a fundamental human requirement. It is critical to health and psychological well-being (Perrin, 1995).

Yet what is the characteristic activity of those with dementia? Inactivity! Doing nothing or sleeping prevail. Bowie & Mountain (1993) reported that, in long-stay care, nearly 87 per cent of the time was spent in apparently purposeless movement, inappropriate behaviour or simply doing nothing. As Briscoe (1990) noted, 'Involvement in enjoyable and meaningful activities is often minimal for the dementia sufferer.' We fail to provide activity in areas not only to do with functional performance, but as Perrin (1995) says '"how to make happy" ... 'My concern is now more to do with the client's being, rather than doing'. Yet how often do we observe joy and engagement in occupation?

If it is unthinkable for you to spend hour after hour staring at the wall exposed to little other than a fluorescent light and bemusing background noise, why should such a malign process be appropriate to the needs of people with dementia? Living in seriously impoverished environments results, not only in psychological ill-being, but in actions that others find irritating as they 'hoard' or 'potter with purpose' in the course of meeting their need for occupation.

Social and Human Contact Needs

We are social creatures. All people need human contact. Intellectual status is irrelevant for 'the desire and ability to make contact with another human being are still very much intact' (Crimmens, 1995). It is crucial to well-being. Social ties have even been found to exert a protective effect against psychological distress. Yet, as with occupation, social needs are often neglected. Isolation is the norm for those with dementia. It is not that we simply fail to engage them in conversation, as for many the ability to converse and understand speech will have been lost, but we actually deny them our presence. The need for human contact may be met by eye contact, a smile in passing or by just sitting alongside somebody, even though nothing is said.

In communal care settings they are in close contact with people who are in their eyes unlike themselves and so these can rarely be their new friends. To compound their isolation, as they cease to behave like the person who has been known for years, established family relations are strained and friendships end. Relationships with professional carers are remote, characterised by social distance and are often task-centred. To illustrate this neglect of the person, as a result of death and admission to hospital, within a period of months there may be a complete turnover of residents within a dementia care unit. Yet nothing will change. As new clients are admitted care routines and task-driven relationships carry on as before. That is how little they mattered. Their presence had no social impact, and neither has their departure. For a person with dementia there is rarely any feeling of 'belonging'.

To be denied human contact may result in the quest for social fulfilment. They may call out, attempt to get out or follow others – behaviours that are intrusive and, for those who are being 'trailed', suffocating.

The Need to Know

Curiosity impels much of what we do. A hunger that characterises the human condition is to find answers to the question: why? We need to know what is going on, who said what to who, what is going to take place next, why something happened? From the moment we see babies fascinated by fingers and toes to the time we see ourselves enquiring what happened, what is wrong, or desperate to know the twists and turns of a storyline, or why we are stuck in a traffic jam, we appreciate how important knowledge is. It is possible that our species is successful because we are so curious. We are driven to know.

Berlyne (1960) coined the term 'epistemic behaviour' or knowledge-augmenting behaviour. It is suggested that not knowing sets up a state of emotional tension which is diminished by seeking knowledge. Curiosity results in exploration of the environment and efforts to acquire information. In their world of not knowing, could this be an explanation for behaviour labelled as wandering? Berlyne (1966) observed early investigatory behaviours that involve some sort of manipulation that changes the unfamiliar object: picking it up, tearing it apart, and so on. How reminiscent are these actions of apparently incomprehensible and, at times, destructive behaviours in dementia. How often do we see people with dementia stroking their clothes, fiddling with objects or plucking carpets and bedclothes? Their world is a strange and unknown place. The ravages of perceptual disturbance in general, and agnosia in particular, the destruction of memory and reasoning transform so much that was once known into mysterious phenomena. Seeing is the application of knowledge and, with so little known, strangeness reigns. So much of what is seen is a pattern without meaning: a puzzle to be investigated and possibly guessed at. For most of the time people with dementia are uncertain of where they are and what is going on around them. To find their way around and avoid being lost in a world of chaos, they attempt to seek meaning.

Their actions, however, may be misinterpreted and seen as challenging. It is not surprising that a number are said to eat inedible objects and place inappropriate items in their mouth. It is doubtful, however, whether many are actually engaged in the act of consumption. Instead they are seeking to 'know'. The most primitive way of finding out is to use the tongue and lips. This is what we see infants do. How often do we read on the packaging of toys that contain small parts, 'Not to be given to children under 36 months of age'. Why? Because we know that curiosity will lead them to place the pieces in their mouths and unwittingly risk choking. What is acknowledged when seen in an infant is not so easy to understand when observed in an aged adult with dementia.

So a person with dementia may seek and manipulate objects in an effort to understand their world and, in the process, may be misunderstood. Yet, when their cognitive destruction is so advanced they no longer understand their own bodily functions, their behaviour may degenerate to a state that other people see as degrading. Very few who smear faeces are doing so to be maliciously destructive. Most are simply correcting the consequences of their own curiosity. A woman living alone eventually finds her way to the toilet. Slowed by age, dexterity affected by arthritis, co-ordination of clothing damaged by dressing apraxia, she finds herself sitting on the toilet with her clothes unknowingly rucked up beneath her. As she opens her bowels she feels increasingly uncomfortable and with her impaired judgement and impoverished reasoning she commits an act that she would never have previously done. To investigate why she feels so uncomfortable she places her hand within her clothing, and on its removal it is covered in faeces. It is foul and disgusting. She attempts to remove it by wiping or shaking it off. Within a short passage of time, however, the fading of the memory trace results in the fragmentation of experience. The act has not been committed. She still feels uncomfortable and, as if for the first time, and to this woman the subjective reality is that it is, she places her hand behind her. The cycle of misfortune commences and unfolds. Each investigation and subsequent attempt to remove the faeces results in what we see as smearing. To her she was just seeking an answer to her own discomfort.

Egocentric Needs

Egocentric needs refer to psychological imperatives such as self-respect, self-determination and control, and a sense of possession ('mine') and, when these are violated or not respected, feelings of anger, jealousy, embarrassment and guilt.

When considering these psychological needs the immediate impression may be one that suggests these are needs acquired in mature adulthood and, as such, destined to be eroded early in dementia. This is not so. While the behavioural 'fine-tuning' is observed in maturity (such as the desire to accumulate wealth and taking pride in one's appearance), we remain in the realm of basic need. These essential needs enable parents to partake in toilet training of their young child by distinguishing desired behaviour and appealing to a sense of achievement and pride ('There's a good boy/girl'). Egocentric needs account for the child's independent will in the third year of life, when they forcefully express self-determination. It is the reason for squabbling when one takes from another and the structure of parallel play between infants breaks down. While the inclination to share has yet to develop, the motivation to possess is already established.

Unsurprisingly, we observe challenging behaviour that is the consequence of failing either to acknowledge or to meet egocentric needs. We have already considered the embarrassment of Patrick (p51), yet we also gain insights into the behaviour of those who parcel and hide faeces, refuse to acknowledge errors and failings, hoard and collect, and refuse to co-operate with those who wish to help. Their conduct cannot simply be reduced to absent-mindedness and a loss of self-awareness.

Sexual Need

There is no age at which sexual activity abruptly ends. For older people, sexual interest and capacity to enjoy sex are not lost (Stokes, 1992). Sexual behaviour may be less frequent, but for many it remains a satisfying experience. Yet this is not the cultural expectation. As a consequence, working with older adults with dementia who demonstrate their sexual need may be prejudiced by our misconception of sexuality in later life.

While the frequency of unacceptable sexually explicit behaviours is relatively low, when difficulties arise these have a disproportionate impact on the capacity of both family and professional carers to cope. Yet our concerns must not be founded on the premise that it is the sexual need which is unacceptable. It is the behaviour that is a problem, not the sexual drive. People with dementia, both young and old, remain sexual beings like ourselves (Archibald, 1995). Then again, are we even sure that the behaviour that is being labelled as an explicit act is of a sexual nature. As was noted earlier (p17) non-sexual actions may be misinterpreted and mistakenly labelled. This is the starting point: *pinpoint* the behaviour and determine whether it is sexual. If it is, then we must establish 'is it a problem' and, if it is, 'for who'? This applies to all challenging behaviours: who is being distressed or disturbed by the actions? Yet in many ways these considerations are most pertinent in the realm of sexual behaviour, the reason being that perception and judgement may be significantly affected by ageist attitudes, or by beliefs that a person with a disability must be asexual. When such prejudices are addressed, the expression of sexuality may no longer be seen as a problem, but as a positive aspect of a person's life.

If the behaviour remains challenging, say we are confronted with public masturbation or fondling of carers or vulnerable others, we must accept the degree to which we are culpable for the onset and maintenance of the unwanted conduct (see Figure 6.1). It is not the sexual need that is deviant, but the expression. Yet what are the acceptable and available outlets of sexual need for a person with dementia? What is available for the man in a residential home, bereft of memory, understanding and reasoning, who is sexually active? If the answer is nothing, then it is to be expected that his sexual need will take him down the path of unacceptable behaviour. To this extent we are culpable. We cannot deny being party to the frustration of what is a human need. Certainly, the destruction of his cognitive powers, losses that distort perception and understanding and lay the foundations for confusion play a significant role in the genesis of his sexual misconduct, but that does not absolve us of all responsibility. We are not working with sexual disinhibition. He cannot be blamed. The sexual drive is normal and our contribution to its unwanted expression cannot be denied. We ignore the fact that we do little or nothing to address or compensate for the frustration of this powerful and fundamental need, then throw up our hands in horror

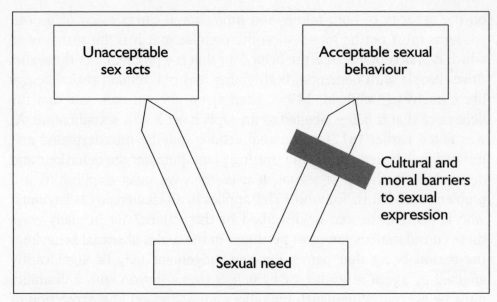

Figure 6.1 *The expression of sexual need in dementia*

when a 'sexual problem' is confronted and protest that 'something must be done'. Yet maybe we do this because we feel that in the real world of care little can be done to meet this need and so we hope that the challenge will never appear. When it does we are ill-equipped to respond with sensitivity and understanding.

Conclusion

Satisfaction and well-being will only be attained when we address meaningfully the needs of those with dementia, needs which are common to all people, yet may be heightened by the experience of dementia (Kitwood, 1997). A subjective world of motivation that cannot be addressed by simple attendance to basic physical needs.

While the nature of need in dementia and the patterns of behaviour that evolve are matters for continuing empirical observation and debate, no longer can we assert that, when cognitive functioning fails us, all that is left is our physical self.

CHAPTER 7
Taxonomies of Possible Explanations

THE PERSON-CENTRED MODEL OF DEMENTIA is, in itself, challenging. A paradigm shift has occurred that enables the finding of solutions. We enter a world where the language resonates with objectives such as understanding, achieving potential, rehabilitation and resolution. However, the penalty is that of complexity. The previous chapters have revealed the richness of explanation. Now the task is to assess and interpret the explanatory pathways. The way they interact has to be appreciated. As a consequence, we need to avoid a sense of being overwhelmed by the volume of information available and then in turn seeking sanctuary in the seductive simplicity of the medical model. To achieve this goal we require methodologies of analysis that bring structure and order to our search for explanation. The first of these is to develop *taxonomies of possible explanations* and learn the benefits of *creative brainstorming*.

Potential Explanations
Ethological research over the past 15 years has provided us with possible explanations when faced with major challenging behaviours that lend themselves to categorisation. In day care, residential and hospital settings, as well as in a person's own home, observation of those with dementia, watching the actions of carers, talking to both caregivers and

those who need to be cared for, has yielded rich data on the possible reasons for behaviour labelled as demanding and difficult. Information that was the driving force behind the development of the person-centred model of understanding, originally referred to as the Multiple Pathway to Behaviour (Stokes & Allen, 1990).

Following on from the assessment practice of defining and pinpointing, we now consider what are the most common explanations for the main challenging behaviours.

Aggression

Defensive behaviour Aggression may be a defensive reaction to threatening intrusion of personal spaces. Providing assistance in basic self-care tasks may be resisted as the purpose is not understood and carers are not recognised. The interrelated issues are the following:

- entering an individual's personal space without invitation or explanation (or if one is provided it is not repeated, and so falls victim to the fragmentation of experience);
- invariably delivering 'hands on', intimate care once in their personal space to a person who is unable to know their dependency needs; and
- failing to acknowledge that we are obscured by a mist of disorientation. Our intentions are unknown and our credibility is minimal, for, while we know who we are and what we are doing, they rarely, and then only fleetingly, ever do.

The outcome has been referred to as 'aggressive resistance' (Hope *et al*, 1997).

Failure of competence With insight remaining, attempts to help the person with activities of daily living may be unwelcome. They are explicit evidence of incompetence and, therefore, help may be resisted and abuse may dominate the attempted episode of care.

Similarly, during assessment, questions designed to test memory and orientation may be met with extreme annoyance and an abrupt termination of the interview. It is understandable that people will not wish to expose their failings or dependence on others as they try to hold onto a conviction that 'all is well'.

Reality confrontation Exposing a confused person to the painfulness of a present which is characterised by a loss of persons, places and things can result in anger and abuse as they live and know a reality of years ago – a response that will be all the more vociferous and violent as others, exhausted and exasperated, lose sensitivity and become 'brutal' in the way they convey information that 'is not true'.

Alarm Abrupt and rapid approaches towards a vulnerable person, possibly poorly sighted and hard of hearing, as well as disoriented, especially if coming from behind or involving unexpected physical contact, can easily result in a hostile act of self-protection.

Misunderstanding events Trying to make sense of an uncertain and mysterious world can easily result in misunderstanding and inappropriate actions. For example, a disoriented man may believe the district nurse who visits his frail wife may be assaulting her; a homecare worker may be regarded as an unwelcome intruder, or a woman on a long-stay ward may hold a belief that fellow patients should respect her privacy and go home. Such misunderstanding can, understandably, be responsible for aggressive actions.

Manipulation In the beginning, when a person retains the cognitive capacity to reason and recall, aggression may be used as a means to manipulate others in order to get their own way. In the absence of the necessary intellectual and memory abilities, this explanation is highly improbable.

Psychosis Aggression has been linked to delusional ideation. In one study it was observed that people with dementia who experienced delusions were four times more likely to be at least mildly aggressive (Gormley *et al*, 1998). It does not appear that hallucinations are related to aggressive acts.

Attention seeking Even though violent behaviour and threatening gestures are uncommon (for example, Hamel *et al*, 1990), when they occur those affected are understandably watchful and ill-at-ease. As a result, it is a powerful means of gaining attention. However, the factors we need to consider when deciding whether 'manipulation' is the reason for aggressive behaviour are also relevant to this potential explanation.

Adaptive paranoia This example of verbal aggression is not evidence of psychosis. Blaming others is a means by which the frightening implications of a deteriorating memory are denied. Making accusations against others to explain why items cannot be found or why an arrangement was forgotten can provide external sources of blame for internally caused mistakes. As such attempts to hide incompetence are early rather than late features of dementia, the accusations may at first appear plausible. Given the risk of older adult abuse and the tendency for others to disempower those with dementia, it is unwise, however, to automatically assume that accusations of maltreatment are without substance.

Goal frustration Aggression may be the reaction to a carer's response to confine or control the drives and desires of those with dementia. Giving instructions to stop or to act differently may provoke an aggressive gesture, as will physical restraint. A person who wanders away from the house or is entering the rooms of others may react with hostility when prevented from doing so. Or maybe it happens when a woman tries to live her home life as she has always done, but unwittingly attempts to put cartons of milk in the oven. Physically preventing such hazardous conduct may result in her 'lashing out, and thrashing me with a tea towel' (the words of a desperate husband). In some people the unwillingness to comply with instructions presents as a wilful attempt to do the opposite of what is requested. This is consistent with the 'age of negativism' observed at the beginnings of selfhood.

During self-care tasks a person may become frustrated and angry because apraxia interferes with the voluntary control of movements. Apraxias are disorders of co-ordination that are not the result of physical or sensory deficits. The person appreciates what to do, but the moment the actions come under conscious control they experience difficulties. The outcome is a marked impairment of daily living skills (the case of Jack, p186). The result is frustration and the potential for unwelcome, but well-meaning assistance, which may in turn be resisted.

Similarly, a person may experience the frustration of being unable to communicate their needs, because speech is affected by expressive aphasia. Frustration-related anger can be compounded when others who are trying to piece together what is being said arrive at obscure interpretations, to the exasperation of the person who is struggling to make themselves understood. The listener's mistaken reasoning is that, if what the person wished to say was simple and straightforward, the words would be produced. As this is not happening, the person must be trying to articulate a complex communication and hence their attempts to 'fill in the gaps' drift into the obscure and irrelevant.

Some researchers (such as Hamel *et al*, 1990) have raised the possibility that a person is more likely to respond aggressively when faced with frustrating situations if their pre-morbid way had always been to do so. While this may account for a proportion of hostile incidents, on many occasions the abuse and aggressive posturing appear 'out of character'.

Impulsive over-reaction An unexpected change of routine, a misplaced article of value or a name that cannot be recalled may result in a poorly controlled outburst of temper, or possibly even rage, as a result of frontal lobe brain damage.

With only a few exceptions there is great aetiological value in knowing the setting in which aggression arises. Researchers (for example, Ware et al, 1990; Gormley et al, 1998) have observed aggressive behaviour occurring most often during intimate care, when responding to instructions or in response to the aggressive acts of others.

Toileting Difficulty
When a person is found 'wet', it is essential to discriminate between incontinence and unsuccessful performance following recognition of the need to urinate.

Incontinence A person may wet themselves owing to failure or impairment of bladder control, so that involuntary voiding occurs. Such dysfunction may arise as a result of the following:

- a localised anatomical or physical abnormality. Incontinence may result from local disorders of the urinary tract. The manner of clinical presentation may result in a diagnosis of stress incontinence (involuntary loss of urine that occurs on physical exertion), urge incontinence (involuntary loss of urine associated with an uncontrollable desire to void which has not been anticipated) or overflow incontinence (the retention of urine with involuntary overflow). Consideration should also be given to the problems of urinary tract infection and constipation;
- secondary nocturnal enuresis. After many years of complete control a person may experience bed wetting at night. This may be attributable to sleep weakening effective bladder control, or it may indicate a more serious condition, such as heart failure;
- loss of bladder control. Incontinence can arise directly from the loss of learned bladder control as a result of cortical atrophy. The outcome can be continuous incontinence. Incontinence may appear relatively early in the course of Pick's disease, as well as in subcortical dementia caused by normal pressure hydrocephalus and multiple sclerosis.

Inappropriate urinating is characterised by an awareness of a need to urinate which does not result in the acceptable voiding of urine.

Neuropsychological dysfunction
- Expressive aphasia will interfere with a person's capacity to communicate their need to urinate, and thus a request for assistance to stand or locate the toilet may flounder on the rock of their disintegrated 'dementia speech'.
- Receptive aphasia (an inability to understand what is being said) will mean that requests to toilet or a query as to whether a person requires assistance may not be understood and hence the need will remain unacknowledged.
- Visual agnosia is a disorder of recognition that results in an inability to identify an object, such as a toilet, by vision alone. Similar objects, such as a wash basin or bath, may be used instead. A man I knew would urinate against white surfaces, including radiators, the side of

a bath and in the corner of a room. A variation is spatial agnosia. This is an inability to find one's way around even familiar places. It looks like disorientation but it is not produced by memory impairment. Unilateral visual inattention or one-side neglect results in a person not 'seeing' anything normally to their left (Holden, 1995). As a result, they will bump into things and fail to see objects. The implications for toileting are easy to appreciate.

- Apraxias interfere with toileting performance. Ideational apraxia means that a person cannot perform a complex task involving a series of movements. Order and sequencing are lost once the action is under voluntary control and the task becomes 'completely disordered' (ibid). With dressing apraxia, attempts to dress result in disorganised actions as the person fails to relate clothing appropriately to their body. A consequence is that it renders the person well nigh incapable of achieving the appropriate arrangement of clothing prior to toileting. The result is soiled and wet clothing.

Disorientation Toileting difficulties can arise following a move to new surroundings. A person who is unfamiliar with their environment may roam around the building searching for the toilet until they are compelled to urinate inappropriately. It does not matter how often they are told, they will never learn, for their inability to store information works against the acquisition of information. Even when a person has lived for many years in the same house the ravages of Ribot's law will result in the person with dementia becoming disoriented as their recent memories are lost.

Environment-dependent Even when a person with dementia is aware of the location of the toilet, the design and layout of the building may make reaching the toilet difficult. The outcome of the 'race' between bladder and legs may depend on the distance which has to be covered and the strength and confidence the aged person possesses to avoid obstacles which may bar the way. Obstacles that may be obvious, such as stairs, steps and heavy doors, and those that may be not, for example non-slip shiny floors that look wet and slippery to a pair of aged eyes, or a pattern on the floor or carpet that may suggest a step or even be seen as 'crawling with worms' (the case of Jane, see p000).

Loss of goal-directed behaviour A person with dementia may get out of their chair with the objective of using the toilet, but then forget what they had intended to do. The fragmentation of experience may leave them walking apparently aimlessly, with no obvious motive, until the urge is so great that they urinate wherever they may be.

Mobility and dexterity Toileting difficulties may be the indirect consequence of physical disability. Despite being able to recognise the need to use the toilet, a person with dementia may be prevented from doing so because of unsteadiness while walking or standing, or because of slowness in moving. Alternatively, the person may reach the toilet in time but have problems opening the door or adjusting their clothing because fine hand movements are compromised by the effects of arthritis or tremor associated with Parkinson's disease.

Depression The appearance of a toileting difficulty may be the result of clinical depression. Older people with dementia are many more times more likely to suffer from depression than those who are not, maybe by a factor of ten. Contrary to belief, loss of insight offers no protection. It is now widely accepted that depression in dementia demands vigorous treatment (Baldwin, 1997). When depressed, loss of interest, poor concentration, apathy and withdrawal combine to interfere seriously with toileting performance.

Apathy Continence is an acquired habit, the motivation for which may diminish with loss of strength and stamina in old age. As life becomes effortful, older adults conserve energy. For a minority, this may result in a disinclination to toilet appropriately.

Fear A person with dementia may be frightened of falling, entering the unknown, negotiating stairs or becoming lost. It does not matter that we assess them as being competent, if a person feels frightened then that is what matters. Fear comes from within and is often impervious to the reassuring words of others. Fear may be exaggerated by sensory impairment.

Embarrassment Being too embarrassed to ask, fearful of humiliation if they were to wet themselves on the way to the toilet, may result in a person discreetly wetting themselves, for inappropriate urinating is the only invasive behaviour that can be committed in 'silence'. Unfortunately, their attempts to preserve dignity may result in condemnation and inevitable embarrassment. In advanced dementia, embarrassment may result in parcelling.

Curiosity This explanation is especially pertinent at times of abnormal bowel movements, for example constipation and diarrhoea, and may account for faecal smearing (see p11). Feeling uncomfortable, the person with dementia investigates to find out why. Having got faeces on their hands, they endeavour to clean themselves and remove the evidence of their actions. The fragmentation of experience and their enduring discomfort maintain their dysfunctional quest for knowledge.

Self-determination The desire to exercise agency in intimate self-care may be so strong as to result in valiant, albeit unsuccessful, attempts to demonstrate independence or a refusal either to ask for, or to accept, assistance.

Manipulation, attention seeking and spite The purpose of inappropriate toileting is to exercise a negative affect on another person. The motivation is to get one's own way, attract attention or retaliate. As cognitive capacity is required to set such objectives, this explanation is only valid at the beginnings of dementia and invariably provides evidence of dysfunctional relationships.

Inadequate facilities In communal arrangements (for example, day centres, residential homes or hospital wards) the number of toilets available may be inadequate to meet the needs of those who are required to use them. This is especially pertinent at times of peak demand, say following mealtimes. The toilets may be difficult to enter, unclean or smell of stale urine; they may be poorly lit or lack adaptations to make them safe; or they may be too public. On their own, these failings do not result in inappropriate toileting. They do, however, discourage use and, as a result, they build in delay as the person embarks upon a potentially fruitless search for an acceptable toilet. The outcome is episodes of wetting and soiling.

Over-dependency Over-concern by a family carer or the de-skilling effects of 'disempowerment' may lead to the premature loss of independent will and a regression to 'infantile' dependency.

Drug effects Toileting difficulties may be a sign of drug side-effects. For example, they may be attributable to excessive drowsiness caused by tranquillisers, or an unwanted response of a person to diuretics. Bed wetting at night may arise following the prescription of night-time sedation.

As can be seen, toileting difficulties are by no means straightforward problems to understand. Motivation and action will also be enshrined within a person's biography (remember Mrs O, pp78–80) and influenced by personal habit (the case of Mrs S, pp52–3). The range of explanation will also be affected by the progression of the presumptive disease. For example, motivational factors will be in part dependent on cognitive competence. Does the person possess insight? To what extent can they retain and recall experience and exercise reason?

It is also the case that identification of cause may be hindered by the hidden nature of the behaviour. It can be difficult to identify accurately an incident of 'wetting' at the time of its occurrence if, for example, the person is either discreet, indifferent or unaware of their bodily functions. There is no simple solution to this difficulty. We need to be especially observant during the pursuit of understanding and heed the clues that come from pinpointing the behavioural characteristics (for example, parcelling – embarrassment; passive wetting – incontinence, depression or fear; smearing – curiosity; active wetting – apraxia, disorientation or poor mobility; inappropriate receptacle – agnosia).

Finally, and this applies to all conduct that is challenging, a person's behaviour is not only unique to them, but can occur at different times for different reasons. To gain a genuine understanding of a person's behaviour it needs to be understood as it is occurring *now*. The case of

Wendy (Box 7.1) illustrates how the reasons for a previous episode of toileting difficulty may have little bearing on the explanation for this or the next challenging incident.

Box 7.1 The trials of Wendy, aged 47 years, a woman with chronic-progressive multiple sclerosis

Wendy's husband could cope with much, but her wetting and soiling was beyond the pale. He would regularly ask whether she needed the toilet, invariably to be told 'no' or to be met with silence. Then some time later she would be found with clothes soiled, or there would be urine and faeces in the bed or on the toilet floor. Her rejection of his help angered him, yet what really infuriated him was that, at the day centre, her toileting difficulties were less severe. Her actions at home seemed deliberate. One day, having found his wife soiled on the way to the lavatory, just moments after asking her whether she needed the toilet, he flew into a rage and grabbed hold of her. The casualty officer's report documented two broken fingers and a dislocated thumb.

There was no single reason for Wendy's behaviour, instead there were reasons, some of which she found impossible to articulate.

- Damaged sphincter control. Incontinence is a common feature of multiple sclerosis, and at times Wendy failed to acknowledge her need to toilet.
- Fatigue. Tiredness and loss of stamina significantly interferes with efficiency in daily life. Wendy would spend much of her time lying on the bed, too tired to respond to her responsibilities and needs.
- Physical limitations on movement. Wendy had lost the sight in one eye and suffered from weakness and spasticity on her right side. As a result her movements were slow and her co-ordination was poor.
- Exaggerated forgetfulness. Wendy's dementia is mild, yet sufficient to compromise her memory and concentration. When somewhere new, she would sometimes struggle to locate the toilet even when reminded.
- Depression. The most frequently observed emotional disturbance in multiple sclerosis is low mood. Wendy's family doctor had been treating her for depression for nearly two years, with little success.

- Forlorn attempts to maintain independence. Wendy is proud. She is determined to maintain her self-respect, even though her physical weakness renders her increasingly dependent and likely to fail.
- Spite. Marital tensions pre-exist Wendy's multiple sclerosis. As her husband continued to live his life, often leaving her alone in the evening, she would retaliate by soiling when he was out. This also enabled her to exercise a degree of control over her husband's activity.
- Embarrassment. In the absence of love and tenderness she found personal care at the hands of her husband awkward and embarrassing. She would rather try herself than experience the indignity of revealing her intimate needs to him.

Repetitive Questioning

Even a seemingly straightforward behaviour such as repetitive questioning requires a thorough understanding of cause. When discussing stressful challenges faced by families, 'demandingness' is regularly cited. Constantly asking questions may be seen as 'deliberate' attempts to inconvenience or upset, or as an example of a lack of concern for the family carer as they seek moments of peace and quiet. Relationships can become so strained that tempers are barely controlled. Care staff are reduced to ignoring or blaming the person. They are driven to respond with 'How many more times must I tell you?' or they despair of answering: 'What's the point? They never remember'. These are clear examples of 'disparagement'.

Short-term memory impairment Marked alterations in a person's ability to store experience can lead to repeated requests for information. Having been heard, within moments the information is lost, and the person is motivated to ask again. As memory worsens, it is not only answers that are forgotten, but the entire experience. The question has never been asked.

Perseveration Repetition may be the result of perseveration. This sign of frontal lobe damage means that questions, words and ideas are repeated continually. This is otherwise known as the 'stuck needle syndrome'. The person cannot shift from what is being asked and so repeats the question again and again. If perseveration is the explanation, the person will get stuck on many occasions and repeat actions as well as words and statements.

Boredom Deprived of occupation and appropriate stimulation, a person with dementia may indulge in repetitive questioning as a means of gaining relief from boredom.

Human contact The person may ask the same question again and again as a means of holding onto the presence of another. It is not the content of the question that is significant, but the achievement of human contact.

Receptive aphasia This is sometimes referred to as Wernicke's aphasia (Holden, 1995). A main feature is an inability to understand what is being said, so what is received is meaningless. While social responses are normal and speech flows, content is often characterised by neologisms, jargon, perseveration, anomia (word-finding difficulties), circumlocution (roundabout explanations and descriptions) and echolalia (echoing). Questioning presents as automatic with minimal intent. Our responses are not understood, so the question is repeated. This explanation is likely if the main features of receptive aphasia are observed in everyday conversation.

Hard of hearing The root of the problem could be as straightforward as not hearing what was said. So many people with dementia are considered to be more forgetful then they truly are, simply because their partial deafness has not been taken into account.

A need for security A person may repeat themselves not solely to keep the company of another but to gain a sense of security. By asking the same question they are able to 'cling' to the reassuring presence of that person. Again the content of the question is of little consequence. It is the hidden message we are required to address.

A forlorn attempt to communicate need Here the content is significant. The question is repeated, not because the answer has been forgotten, but because the need remains unmet. Our response may have been to correct, believing their questioning represents confusion. Yet as we saw in Chapter 4, what is said may represent the communication of need, a need that we fail to acknowledge. For example, consider the possible reasons for repetitively asking the following:

- Where are my children? (The articulation of a need to be loved and needed.)
- Where is my wife? (Communication of a need to be secure or a need for intimacy.)
- Where is my mother? (Communication of a need to be comforted and reassured.)
- When can I go home? (A desire to be safe, or possibly an expression of the physical need to toilet.)

Even a question such as 'When's dinner?' may convey messages, not only 'I'm hungry', but the articulation of a need to be secure. Mealtimes are when families eat together. Parents, partners and children are present. It is the security that eating together brings which is being communicated.

As we pass them by, offering little other than correction and 'matter of fact' information, they repeat the question again and again.

Wandering
Having appreciated that we all, regardless of intellectual status need to walk, if a person's behaviour does fall within the operational definition of wandering there is no single explanation to account for the behaviour, the reason being that, as with other challenging behaviours, wandering does not constitute a coherent syndrome. Instead, there are different types of wandering, each of which has its their own explanation. If we refer to the behavioural characteristics (see p32), a person who 'potters with purpose', is unlikely to indulge in 'exit behaviour' or 'trailing and tracking', for each is the behavioural consequence of a different motivation. Unless needs change, other wandering 'characteristics' are unlikely to appear, and rarely will we observe simultaneous expression unless the actions share a common motivational bond.

Separation anxiety When in the company of another whose presence provides reassurance and peace of mind, all is *relatively* well. Unfortunately, as that person lives their life, they move around the house, or go out. The fragmentation of experience means that there is no recollection of where they have gone, how long they have been away, or any message to the effect that they will return. They are just absent. Separation anxiety motivates those with dementia to cling to this other person ('trailing and tracking') or, if the person with dementia is removed to another setting in order to give their family respite from the suffocating pressure of being 'trailed', they will attempt to leave in order to seek those significant others ('attachment behaviour').

Confusion An attempt to find somebody who, or something which, no longer exists for it resides in their past. Searching for young children, going home and seeking deceased loved ones, usually parents or a spouse, are common motivations. Their determination to 'search for their past' is borne out of conviction and invariably does not benefit from reality orientation. To us their walking is directed towards an inappropriate goal, but that is not how it is to them.

Habits of a lifetime People with dementia may indulge in actions that are confused continuations of what they have always done. These 'comfortable remnants' are now inappropriate to context: for example, walking around at night, 'securing' the residential home before going to bed. We observed occupational remnants when understanding the actions of Emily and Horace (p72).

Living life As people with dementia carry out the practical tasks of daily life and pursue comfortable behaviours, the pursuit of these appropriate goals may be intrusive. The person may become a nuisance if the task is carried out with inappropriate frequency (for example, watering houseplants throughout the day; visiting the post office hour-after-hour; checking to see if the front door is closed) or they may cause concern, for they are no longer able to appreciate danger or know that they will become lost. The challenge to others may be that the motivation is inappropriate at the time chosen ('appropriate goal, inappropriate time').

Examples would be going to the shops when they are closed, leaving to visit relatives in the early hours of the morning or attempting to walk in the garden during the hours of darkness.

Physical discomfort As walking can ease discomfort, and even distract us from our suffering, a person with dementia may start to walk around. As they are unable to articulate a reason for their excessive activity, we see 'apparently aimless' or 'restless' movement.

Coping with stress To pace is a stress response ('the caged animal', 'the expectant father'). Some people go for a walk when they are troubled. These are further explanations for 'restless pacing'.

Failure of navigation An inability to store new experiences or recall previously learned information will result in a person becoming lost within a building as they try to locate, for example, their bedroom or the toilet ('place disorientation').

Boredom Inactivity motivates a person with dementia 'to do'. As they walk around busying themselves, their actions are purposeful, even though the observed actions may be bizarre, for example gathering others' possessions, moving furniture or manipulating objects. While their wandering may be a nuisance to us, 'pottering with purpose' is a source of contentment. If their 'pottering' is reminiscent of known patterns of behaving, it is categorised as a 'comfortable behaviour', possibly a historical remnant.

Loneliness The person with dementia who lives alone may leave their home to find companionship. The motivation is not inappropriate, the challenge is that they do not appreciate the risks involved ('walking with risk towards an appropriate goal') or the appropriate purpose is repeated to excess ('over-appropriate behaviour'). In communal settings, it is not that they are isolated, but 'being alone in a crowd' motivates them to walk around in an effort to find a friendly face to be with. This may result in 'following behaviour'.

Curiosity A person may wander as they search for meaning and answers. We observe 'apparently aimless walking', 'exit behaviour' or 'place disorientation'.

Fear In an unfamiliar place, or faced with the strangeness of others, those with dementia may be so frightened that they are desperate to leave ('exit behaviour'). Alternatively, they may roam around unsuccessfully seeking sanctuary. Disorientation may add to their fear.

Avoidance A person who is unable to voice their complaints may seek to escape from unpleasant environmental 'noise'. Suffering the meaningless stimulation of a television, having to endure age-inappropriate background music or the calling out of others can understandably result in their trying to get out and becoming lost, or apparently walking without purpose once the motivation to walk has been forgotten.

Perseveration Frontal-lobe damage may result in walking to excess, for no obvious reason. Perseveration means that their actions are not under voluntary control. Malcolm, a 50-year-old man with probable Pick's disease, does very little other than walk continuously around his home. He has a set route that he follows; through the lounge, along the hall, through the kitchen and back into the lounge. Having completed his circuit many times, he will sit for a few moments before getting up and starting again.

Spatial agnosia Spatial agnosia will make it so difficult for a person to find their way around, even in buildings known well, that they will end up lost as they try to identify 'landmarks' that make sense.

Sundowning Agitated, purposeless wandering or determined exit behaviour may occur at the end of the day. Often known as 'sundowning', this may be the consequence of cellular destruction producing diurnal rhythm disturbance (see p38). On the other hand, it may have psychological roots. From our earliest years we are accustomed to departing as the day ends. We went home from school, we go home from work. Triggered by both internal and external cues, the person with dementia may start to move around in early evening for no apparent reason.

Fragmentation of experience A person may get up with a task or plan in mind, but then forget what they had intended to do, leaving them wandering aimlessly with no apparent motive.

Given the variety of reasons that motivate us to walk, it is hardly surprising that the same richness of motivation underpins a tendency to wander. No longer can it be said that a person with dementia wanders because they have dementia.

Noise Making

Noise making is loud and persistent vocalising, as measured by duration or frequency, which can be either intelligible or unintelligible and is resistant to requests for silence. The behavioural characteristics include yelling, disruptive talk, melodic sounds, calling out and groaning. See also the typology of verbal and vocal disruptive behaviours proposed by Cohen-Mansfield & Werner (1997).

With the move towards care at home and the development of small-scale continuing care units, noise making is a behaviour that can be difficult to tolerate by all involved. Yet it cannot be regarded as a nuisance to be ignored, rebuked or 'isolated'. We need to improve our understanding of the reasons which make a person with dementia indulge in disruptive noise making, even when vocalisations are unintelligible and we have to infer probable cause.

Pain The communication of physical pain and discomfort may result in yelling, calling out or groaning.

Environmental discomfort A person's noise making may be a response to unpleasant conditions. For example, the room in which they are sitting may be too hot or too cold; they may be sitting in the glare of the sun or under stark fluorescent lighting; their chair may be uncomfortable.

Talking to others Their attempts to talk may be 'bothersome' because they are too loud. Loudness may be affected by poor hearing or the unresponsiveness of the person to whom they are 'talking'. This explanation is more likely if distinct words are discernible and the person is directly gazing at somebody.

Needs to be met A person may call out because they have needs to be met. We may hear the most obvious indicator of need – 'help me, help me' – but unintelligible yelling may be a forlorn attempt to communicate that, for example, they are hungry or thirsty, need the toilet or wish to get out of their chair or go to bed.

Psychosis Subject to hallucinations, a person with dementia may talk to or shout at someone who is not present as if they were interacting with an individual who was there.

Under-stimulation Frequent screaming and shouting may be an effort to provide self-stimulation when living a life characterised by inactivity and isolation. Under-stimulation may be compounded by failing eyesight and poor hearing. When environmental and sensory deprivation accounts for noise making, it may be accompanied by repetitive physical movements. Shouting may be most marked at night as the person lies awake during the hours of darkness experiencing silence as an unpleasant source of sensory deprivation. Their apparent disregard for other people is a result of their subjective lack of awareness that there are others.

Abandonment Calling out the name of a loved one, either near and present or unavailable, demonstrates insecurity and the pain of separation. The person with dementia is unable to recall that all is well when regularly reminded, or perhaps reassurance is not possible now that they are living a time long gone. Prosopagnosia, while rare, may promote a sense of abandonment as a person is no longer able to recognise familiar faces. Relatives will be seen as strangers and be able to offer no comfort. The calling out continues.

A stress reaction Agitated shouting can be an indication that the person is distressed. The noisy behaviour may be a fear response, most commonly observed either when sitting alongside somebody whose behaviour is intimidating or at night when the person awakes in surroundings that are mysterious. At such times they may call out for their parents. Alternatively, a person may sing a familiar song or repetitively call out a phrase, as if reciting a mantra in order to experience feelings of reassurance.

Over-stimulation When sitting in a hectic and crowded room, or being bombarded with instructions, a person with dementia may experience an excess of environmental stimulation and resort to either agitated shouting or loud vocalising which introduces into the environment a noise which they are able to control. Busy moments in communal settings, such as mealtimes, may trigger calling out. A caring husband once described how he and his three children were telling his wife why she must stop preparing the meal. She was doing silly things (cooking with saucepans containing no water, the tea towel draped over the hob) and they had visions of imminent disaster. In the midst of this babble of conversation and demands, she just started shouting incoherently. Have you ever felt so swamped by the pressure of others that you could scream? If you are dementing, you may do.

Perseveration Whenever we observe behaviour that is repeated over and over again for no apparent purpose, it is always possible that the person is perseverating.

Attention seeking When possessing the cognitive capacity to manipulate the social environment, noise making may be employed to attract attention. Others understandably attempt to find out what is wrong or try to persuade the person to be quiet. So often it is observed that only at times of disruption is a person with dementia in receipt of social contact. The unintentional consequence is to encourage the behaviour that others wish would not occur.

Noise making can be a major challenge both to families and to professional caregivers. It can be so disturbing that the behaviour easily introduces intolerable strain into the lives of carers. Pressures can be so great that care can break down and requests for a change of placement in the interests of others is a common development. Yet by understanding that we are again working, not with a unitary challenging construct, but with different behavioural phenomena each with different explanations, enables us to move towards specific solutions rather than unwisely concentrating on techniques of management, although, as Cohen-Mansfield & Werner (1997) note, unintelligible noise presents us with the greatest difficulty in attributing meaning.

Creative Brainstorming

Rigorous observation and analysis over several years has borne rich fruit. The taxonomies of possible explanation enable us to understand the complex nature of even the most apparently straightforward challenging behaviours (for example, repetitive questioning). Patient watching and listening succeeded in opening our eyes and ears to a world to which the standard paradigm had failed to make reference. This same quest for understanding can inform and benefit everyday care practice. If we are watchful and creative in our thinking we can brainstorm possible explanations for any behaviour that is challenging. The methodology may lack scientific rigour, but what it brings is a dynamic approach to enquiry. If a person keeps coming out of their room at night, refuses food, climbs into another person's bed, will not walk into a lift, places inedible objects in their mouth or removes their clothes, ask why.

Do not be constrained by dwelling solely on the expected, for if the explanation was so obvious it is likely that it would already have been addressed. The art of successful brainstorming progresses through the following steps:

1   *Generate* as many explanations for the behaviour as possible. Be creative. Use imagination to move beyond the obvious. It does not matter whether ideas are a variation on a theme. Bring colleagues into the exercise. Even involve those who do not know the person or their circumstances, for their contribution will not be tempered by knowledge of the individual and their difficulties. Focus on the improbable. For who knows, it may be within the seemingly unlikely that the reason is to be found. Place yourself in the situation of the person. Demonstrate empathy for their world. The purpose behind creative brainstorming is that it is likely to capture a host of ideas. If, instead, we adopt an incremental approach, painstakingly moving

from the obvious to the less so, we generate little in comparison and rarely arrive at the truly unlikely.

2   *Eliminate* those explanations that beyond all doubt do not apply, where either no enquiry or only minimal discussion is required to determine that the proposed reasons do not pertain to the person, their behaviour or their needs. Many ideas will fall within this category. Those involved in the person's welfare are able to dismiss them with ease. If there is any thought that an explanation might, however unlikely, have some bearing on the nature of a person's difficulties, the explanation cannot be rejected.

3   *Investigate* those ideas that remain. Talk to the person. Gather information by talking to others and asking for health assessments. Build on what is already known about the person to create a pen profile relevant to the current challenge. Walk the building to see if there are design weaknesses. Monitor behaviour to see if a pattern exists (for example, does the behaviour occur at specific times, with certain people, after certain experiences or incidents?) Ask yourself how you would be, what would you do in the same circumstances?

After such enquiry, those explanations that remain viable can be tested. Through a process of 'informed trial and error', address each explanation in turn to see if resolution occurs. We may start with the most likely reason for the behaviour, or possibly one that lends itself to simple remedy. If no change occurs, we move on to the next, until it is hoped the cause is identified and the challenging behaviour can be resolved. What may happen instead is that there is no single cause, but a number of related explanations are revealed, each of which requires intervention.

The following case history illustrated how caregivers working in a residential home used creative brainstorming to resolve the challenge of a man who would not get out of bed. Ian, an unmarried 75-year-old man, had been admitted seven weeks earlier to a specialist dementia care unit. When at home he would get out of bed in the morning either spontaneously or when prompted. Now he would stay in bed, lying silent, rejecting all efforts to help him get up. His behaviour was a problem, causing great concern to staff, for he would lie in his own urine and faeces for hour after hour.

Many ideas were generated by the staff team and these are detailed in Box 7.2. Those marked (*X*) identify the ones eliminated as not warranting investigation. Of the 94 possible explanations proposed, 38 were rejected either immediately or following brief discussion within the group meeting.

Box 7.2 Why won't Ian get up? The use of creative brainstorming to develop understanding

Health

Stroke	(*X*)
Fractured hip	(*X*)
Broken leg	(*X*)
Feeling unwell	
Postural hypotension	
Arthritic pain	
Dizzy	
Oversedated	(*X*)

'Dementia'

Misperception of patterned floor	
Receptive aphasia	(*X*)
Frontal lobe apathy	
Time disorientation – thinks it is night	
Agnosia – makes his world perplexing and threatening	(*X*)

Mobility

Afraid to walk	(*X*)
Unsteady on feet	(*X*)

Personal History

Night-shift worker	(*X*)
Used to having breakfast in bed	
Waiting for a cup of tea before rising	
Waiting to hear newspapers being pushed through letterbox	
Waiting for his dog to bark	(*X*)
Cultural neglect (carers not responding to cultural needs)	
Used to staying in his bedroom	

Sensory

Poor eyesight (X)

Deafness – cannot hear request to get up (X)

Mood and Emotion

Wants to die

Depression

Delusion – being told to stay in bed

Homesick

Frightened

Self

Does not like being taken to the toilet

Protecting his belongings

Fearful of residents

Fears falling

Suspicious of others

Language barrier (X)

Wanting someone familiar to get him up

Does not wish to mix with others

Thinks floor is slippery

Feels safe in bed

Believes someone else may climb into his bed

Enjoys lying there thinking and dreaming

Shy

Dislikes clothes he must wear

Rebelling as does not like being told what to do

Wishes to masturbate in private

Believes it is too early to get up.

Discreetly wetting, as fears he will wet himself while trying
   to locate the toilet

Wishes to dress himself

Comfortable in bed

Wishes to avoid breakfast

Time passes more quickly in bed

Wants to stay in his pyjamas

Enjoys the view (X)

Does not like smoky atmosphere in lounge (X)
Does not like crowded lounge (X)
Wants privacy when dressing
Asserting self-determination
Wants to lie in as believes it is his day off/or on holiday
Believes he is in hospital and so should stay in bed
Too tired – late night (X)
Too tired – disturbed night
Feels nothing to get up for
Does not want a bath (X)
Fearful of water (X)
Apathetic and lazy
Does not like staff
Does not like women caring for him
Does not want to see visitors
Attention seeking
Embarrassed because he is wet
Feels cold
Embarrassed to show his body
Wants to read in bed
Wants to listen to the radio in bed
Waiting for his wife (X)
Hungover (X)
Waiting for someone to ask nicely (X)

Environmental

No clothes to wear (X)
Ill-fitting, uncomfortable clothing (X)
No clean clothes (X)
Inappropriate clothing (eg, style not age appropriate) (X)
Not his own clothes (X)
Floor is cold (X)
Broken cord on pyjamas (X)
Bed too high (X)
No clock to let him know the time (X)
No watch to check the time (X)

Cot sides on the bed are raised	(X)
No slippers	(X)
No dressing gown	(X)
Shoes too tight	
Room too cold	(X)
Room too dark	(X)
Other	
Sponsored lie-in	(X)

Investigation involved the following:

- examination of Ian and review of medication by GP;
- neuropsychological examination and assessment of mood by clinical psychologist;
- talking to his family about Ian – his history and what type of man he is now;
- staff reviewing their approach towards getting Ian out of bed and questioning how they would feel living in the home.

The outcome of the enquiry revealed that Ian was possibly

- depressed;
- wishing to stay in his own room – he would spend a lot of time in his bedroom at home listening to the radio and watching television;
- rebelling – he was always known as stubborn;
- unlikely to welcome women caring for him;
- comfortable in bed;
- avoiding meals and drinks, as he had always been a 'fussy eater', as well as not liking tea and coffee;
- embarrassed if wet – he was known as a proud man.

'Trial and Error' intervention
Before the use of anti-depressants was considered, a commode was placed in Ian's room and he was asked whether he wished to use it every two hours during the day and before sleeping at night. On several occasions,

following a prompt, he would use it independently. However, while he was less likely to be found lying in bed wet and soiled, he was no more likely to get up.

Space was made in his room and an armchair from home (he had been living with his brother and sister-in-law) was placed by the window. This intervention had minimal effect. However, when a television was positioned opposite, and a glass of orange squash was placed next to the chair, Ian would get up with minimal prompting. The final step in resolving Ian's difficulties was to encourage him to walk outside his room to the toilet a little way down the corridor.

The formulation was that Ian felt comfortable and secure in the privacy of his own room and was reluctant to leave. With nowhere to sit (other than on an upright chair) he would lie on his bed. With no en-suite toilet to use, he would discreetly wet and soil himself after getting into bed. Embarrassment then exacerbated his desire to stay there. Providing a commode presented Ian with an accessible toileting facility. With the introduction of an armchair and television there was no reason to lie on the bed and, with the stimulation now on offer, it is likely that his mood lifted. Feeling better 'in himself', Ian was more inclined to respond to prompts and venture outside his room to the toilet. Only rarely, however, would he respond to suggestions to sit in communal areas and mix with others. But that was Ian, a man who enjoyed solitude and watching television.

CHAPTER 8

Behavioural, Ecobehavioural and Functional Analysis

HAVING ESTABLISHED THE COMPLEX ORIGINS of behaviour, systematic and *direct* observation may be very useful in successfully identifying reasons for the appearance and maintenance of a person's disruptive conduct. The objective is to establish whether there is a relationship between the behaviour and its context.

Several methods have been used to observe behaviour, all of which are 'time expensive'. The methodologies all require professional carers to dedicate time to the exercise of reliable observation and recording. This is why, in the real world of care, I often view creative brainstorming as the favoured first step towards achieving accurate understanding. It is nowhere near as time consuming and may lead to early answers. Only if the methodology is unsuccessful, or if we wish to bring precision to our quest for knowledge, are we encouraged to embark upon structured observational techniques.

Observation Schedules

As we are attempting to find out why a person behaves the way they do, we are not concerned with schedules that simply record 'inappropriate' behaviour: for example, the Behavioural Assessment Scale of Later Life (Brooker *et al*, 1993) or the Present Behavioural Examination (Hope &

Fairburn, 1992). Instead we extend the observation format to examine the person–environment interaction. Cohen-Mansfield *et al* (1992) developed the Agitation Behaviour Mapping Instrument to establish the frequency of 'agitated' behaviours. Observers would also record to whom or what the behaviour appears directed, what may have triggered the agitation and what was the reaction of others.

A direct observation method that has become increasingly popular and influential over the past decade is Dementia Care Mapping (DCM) (Kitwood & Bredin, 1992; Fox, 1995). The observational technique of DCM is not specific to challenging behaviour, but examines in general the social psychology of dementia care. The method records the quality of interaction, whether there is evidence of 'personal detraction' (episodes that are demeaning or abusive) and the resulting 'feeling state' of the person with dementia. Fox (ibid) describes how mappers are asked 'to merge gently into the setting' and 'take the standpoint of the person with dementia to gain an empathic sense of what his or her life may be like'. In successive five-minute time frames throughout the period of observation, the mapper records what types of activities and inactivities are occurring and the state of relative well-being or ill-being. As a result, we are able to map out the quality of social interaction and identify incidents and experiences of, for example, disempowerment, inactivity, being ignored, objectification, invalidation, infantilisation, banishment and the accompanying signs of frustration, fear, boredom and emotional distress that others define as challenging.

While DCM should contribute much to our understanding and prevention of challenging behaviour, to date this has yet to be empirically tested (Moniz-Cook, 1998).

Behavioural, Ecobehavioural and Functional Analysis

The rich potential of behavioural analysis has been acknowledged by several specialists in dementia care (for example, Hodge, 1984; Stokes, 1990a; Bleathman & Morton, 1994; Perrin, 1996). In the mid-1980s I described the use of behavioural analysis to examine the relationship between the environment and wandering (Stokes, 1986a), screaming and shouting (Stokes, 1986b), inappropriate urinating (Stokes, 1987a) and aggression (Stokes, 1987b).

Behavioural analysis is often referred to as an ABC analysis: 'A' for activating event or situation (the technical term is 'Antecedents'), 'B' for behaviour, 'C' for consequences. We want to know when the behaviour occurred, where it took place, what was happening at the time and what was the response of others. We are attempting to determine whether the challenging behaviour is triggered by events or being maintained by the consequences of behaving that way, many of which will be social responses. From what we know of dementia, and what was described under the taxonomies of explanation, recall deficits invariably militate against the maintenance of behaviour by a learned appreciation of the consequences that will follow, at least in cases of advanced dementia.

Behavioural analysis is, however, no longer a crude, mechanistic study of the environmental controls of behaviour. It places the person at the centre of our understanding, yet accepts that, as the normal avenues of communication have been denied, we must probe in order to uncover the person and their motivations. It involves using 'such tools as are available, and chipping away at the dross until the nuggets shine through' (Perrin, 1996).

The Process of Behavioural Analysis

Target behaviour The first objective is to determine which challenging behaviour is going to be the focus of analysis. Even if a person is challenging in several domains it is advisable to choose a single behaviour in order that a thorough understanding of the 'target' behaviour is achieved in terms of its environmental setting and the meaning it may possess for the person. Another reason for selecting a single behaviour is that successful resolution may exercise a positive effect above and beyond the chosen intervention in terms of both the person's well-being and the responsiveness of the social environment to their wider needs.

Consideration should also be given to whether the most troublesome behaviour should be the initial target for analysis and potential intervention. To show staff that needs can be met and that as a result behaviour changes, it can be wise to choose a relatively 'soft' target. An apparently minor success can motivate carers and foster a climate of positive expectation.

Behavioural description As we saw in Chapter 2, it is important to provide a precise definition of the target behaviour to be observed and recorded, thereby avoiding 'fuzzy', imprecise statements. To keep personal opinion and interpretation to a minimum, we describe the behaviour in terms of the behavioural boundaries and characteristics. Everybody involved with the person then knows exactly what they are having to monitor, because the definition so carefully detailed is *agreed* by all.

Recording methodology The ABCs are recorded each time an incident is observed, although, as Perrin (1996) notes, it is only in an ideal world that we can observe and record a behaviour throughout the day or night. Instead, we may employ momentary time sampling where a person's behaviour is observed at predetermined points of time. Alternatively, the nature of the behaviour may dictate that we select a specified period each day, say an afternoon or an hour each morning, and record each episode within that time frame. Whatever method is selected, and obviously the greater the length of time or number of observation points, the more accurate the picture revealed, it is essential that (a) all staff are aware that the behaviour is being monitored, and (b) all information is recorded as near to the time of the incident as possible, as it is easy to forget the exact circumstances if recording is left until later.

The collection of information on possible contributory factors can be displayed on a record chart similar to that below.

Day, date, time	Duration	A	B	C	Background

The information on day and time may reveal a temporal pattern (for example, 'sundowning'). For certain behaviours it is not frequency, but duration, which is of most significance, for example: the duration of an episode of noise making, or the length of time of agitated pacing.

The A (activating) column records what was happening immediately before the target behaviour was observed. What had they been doing? What was happening around them at the time? Who was present? If we are confronted with a toileting difficulty, we would need to record answers to the following questions:

- Where were they?
- Had there been a request to toilet?
- Had the person been agitated?
- Had they been observed sitting or walking around?
- What had been happening prior to the incident?
- Who was around them at this time?
- Who was *not* around at this time?

In the B (behaviour) column, we do not simply tick or state 'yes' to demonstrate that behaviour occurred. Instead, we take full advantage of the operational definition and describe precisely what happened by answering the following:

- Where did it occur?
- What did the person do? (Stand or sit passively? Use an inappropriate receptacle?)
- Did they seem aware of their actions?
- Did they appear agitated, distressed or indifferent towards the incident?

The C (consequences) column details what occurs immediately after the incident.

- What was the response of others to the person wetting or soiling themselves?
- What was said to the person?
- Did the person attract the attention of others to the incident?
- What was the person's reaction to the attention of others?
- Did the person attempt to conceal evidence of their toileting difficulty?

The background column covers circumstantial details which enable us to place the immediacy of the ABCs into a broader situational and contextual framework. For example, has anything happened during the day (or night) which may have caused upset? Has there been a recent change in routine, or the introduction of medication? Are the toilet facilities accessible, or difficult to reach or locate? Has there been a recent change in eating behaviour? Is the person drinking more fluids than usual? Has the person recently moved to new surroundings?

If background information is not collected, essential reasons for B occurring, as well as why the person was in situation A, and why they and others reacted at C in the manner they did, will be missed. When we address the context within which behaviour occurs, we are moving into the realm of behavioural ecology. To meet a person's needs it may be the case that a fundamental restructuring of the overall environment is required (Stokes, 1990b). The need to look beyond a limited view of the environment is revealed by the plight of Jack.

Jack was often found wet in the corridors of the residential home (B). Although this could happen throughout the day, it was most frequently observed around mid-morning. Behavioural analysis recorded that, prior to wetting himself, he would be walking around the building agitated and apparently confused (A). He would be demanding to go home and protesting, 'I am fed up with this place, this isn't my home.' His confusion was either ignored or corrected in a cursory manner by passing staff who were busying themselves with household tasks (A). On being discovered wet, staff would at last devote time to him. There was now a task to be done. They would take him to the bathroom to be washed, and then to his bedroom to be changed (C): actions that Jack often resisted.

When it was suggested to staff that they were ignoring Jack's needs, and that his agitated 'confused' behaviour was in fact the actions of a man desperate to communicate his need for the toilet ('I am fed up with this place, this isn't my home. The toilet should be there and it's not, I NEED THE TOILET!') they readily understood. They appreciated that they needed to give him more time, pace their communication and listen to the messages, but the home manager wished all the beds to be made, the residents' rooms to be tidied and the dining tables wiped down before the mid-morning drinks were served at 11.15 (the behavioural context). Only physical care tasks could be accommodated within this schedule. Any suggestion that flowed from the behavioural analysis would inevitably founder on the bedrock of institutional inflexibility, unless an analysis also included an appreciation of the behavioural ecology.

An ecobehavioural analysis (Emerson, 1993) provides an accurate and detailed description in terms of how often the behaviour occurred, the circumstances in which it arose and the consequences for the person, as well as any relevant background features, both situational and contextual.

The procedure The observation and recording of the target behaviours should take place over a period of one to two weeks in order to avoid making decisions on the basis of short-term fluctuations in behaviour. In other words, monitoring for just a few days may result in staff having unwittingly chosen a couple of good days or a particularly bad patch, thereby giving rise to misleading conclusions. Taking time to assess helps avoid unjust labelling and rash decisions. Actions that may not only be unhelpful but lead to even greater challenges.

This stage of behavioural analysis is known as the *baseline period*. It helps to identify not only whether a consistent pattern exists, but also the *frequency* of the challenging behaviour: that is, how many times the target behaviour occurred during the baseline period. Sometimes it is the case that if the challenging behaviour is observed to have a low frequency, this provides evidence that carers have lost perspective (unless the challenge is the duration of the activity, for example, noise making or pacing). Being confronted by a demanding, invasive behaviour can sap energy, erode tolerance and, as a result, appear unremitting. Snyder *et al* (1978) found that even those labelled as 'continuous wanderers' spent much of the time sitting. When the low frequency is discussed with the staff team, they may conclude that the behaviour is not a significant challenge warranting special attention. We continue to consider which needs are unmet at a time of dysfunctional conduct, but such understanding does not require the introduction of extraordinary arrangements.

If a genuine challenge exists, the frequency observed forms the baseline against which future change is measured. Having considered any pattern that is revealed by the analysis, the next step is to respond to the needs of the person, thereby resolving their challenging behaviour. Whatever form intervention may take, the frequency of the target behaviour continues to be recorded so that success can be confirmed or denied, success often being a meaningful reduction in frequency, not the ideal of zero frequency. If there are no positive developments, our formulation was wrong and the intervention requires re-examination. Thus the continued use of frequency recording does away with subjective impressions of whether improvement has occurred or not.

For a detailed and honest account of behavioural analysis, see Perrin (1996).

Functional Analysis

While the collection of ABCs provides us with a detailed description of the relationship between environmental events and behaviour, we cannot restrict ourselves to such a limited methodology. We need to incorporate the multiple determinants of a challenging behaviour and establish its meaningful nature. In other words, we must continue to frame our understanding in accord with the person and their needs. Certainly, a challenging behaviour occurs in a particular setting and it may be inextricably related to that situation and its broader context, but, as we have detailed at length, it is also a function of the person and their motivations. Functional analysis builds on the empirical rigour of a behavioural analysis and addresses the function served by the challenging behaviour. Moniz-Cook *et al* (in press) employed functional analysis to understand five people who were described by staff as 'the most difficult residents to manage in the home', people described as agitated, noisy, demanding, uncooperative and aggressive.

Given our understanding of the person-centred model of dementia it is unsurprising that researchers have identified 'the functional significance of even the most bizarre and serious behaviours' (Samson & McDonnell, 1990). Functional analysis does not restrict itself to an appreciation of the immediate antecedents and/or consequences of a behaviour, but attempts to gain an understanding of the meaning and, possibly, usefulness (that is, the function) 'of a particular behaviour, in a particular set of circumstances, for a particular individual' (ibid). As a result, the pursuit of explanations not only includes that which is observed, but, following a detailed investigation of 'person variables', for example life history, abilities and needs, also addresses the importance of these 'unobservables' (for example, preferences, feelings, individual characteristics, neuropsychological impairment, ill-health or sensory losses). In other words, reference is made to the health and psychogenic pathways (Figure 5.1).

The use of 'unobservables' increases the explanatory power of a functional analysis and helps us achieve an imaginative person-centred explanation. This is a considerable advance on the radical behavioural perspective, which tries to establish relationships between observable behaviour and the observable features of the person's environment, and then attempts to modify behaviour by changing that environment (see Chapter 11) – an approach that is in essence inimical to person-centred dementia care. Let us consider the trials of Mr G (Box 8.1).

Box 8.1 Mr G: a man to be known

Mr G resided in a specialist dementia care unit. He was disoriented, uncommunicative and, at times, intimidating. Sitting in the lounge, he was quiet and withdrawn; that is, until he was either prompted to use the toilet or was being checked to see if he was wet. On these occasions he was abusive, threatening and, on many occasions, violent (B). The antecedents were clear. He was rarely aggressive unless he was subject to intimate care, and behavioural analysis revealed that actions pertaining to toileting (A) were far more likely to invoke a violent response, even though approaches by staff were measured and respectful.

Mr G's violent conduct was not maintained by the consequences of his actions for the reactions of carers were many and varied (C). Most often they persisted with their efforts to toilet him, at other times they would walk away, scold or disparage him. On a few occasions they would attempt to restrain him. The absence of consistent responses suggests that Mr G was not acting the way he did in order to gain a desired reaction.

With regard to situational or contextual features, while the social environment was responsive to the individual toileting needs of clients, both the layout and the interior design of the unit unfortunately left much to be desired. The two toilets were away from the main living area and obscured by ubiquitous magnolia paint. These features clearly exacerbated Mr G's disorientation. However, he never did, and never had attempted to meet his toileting needs. It was probable that his toileting difficulty was not so much environment-dependent, as evidence of embarrassment. He did not know where to go or who to ask, and so he did nothing.

Yet why was Mr G so resistive and violent? How had a man whose family protested he had always been well-mannered, changed so much, transformed to a point where the continuation of his care at the unit was being placed in jeopardy?

Mr G had been a teacher, rising towards the end of his career to deputy headmaster at the school where he had worked for over 27 years. His wife described him as serious, stubborn, conservative in outlook and taciturn. She reflected that he possibly had an undue concern for appearances and, irritatingly, had an inflated sense of his own importance. He did not cope well with setbacks, invariably losing perspective and becoming disillusioned. He enjoyed solitude. His passion outside work was his garden, where he would spend many contented hours. In company, he was ill at ease, unless he clearly knew what was expected of him. Small talk was not for him. Yet his wife impressed upon us that he was always well-meaning, with a concern for others. He would never wish to cause offence. When approached, he would try to be helpful. Yet his manner was often misunderstood, and others rarely warmed to him.

The 'person variables' are clearly fundamental to our understanding of Mr G's violent conduct. The function of his challenging behaviour was to ward off the unwelcome attention of others whose actions were invasive. The motivation for his behaviour was in accord with his known personality, a personality that potentiated the behaviour-environment relationship that the behavioural analysis had identified.

Functional analysis generates many ideas that are not just context-dependent, but most importantly are specific to the person. Moniz-Cook *et al* (in press) found that in spite of the similarity of their challenging behaviours, both the hypothesised person variables to which their actions were related and the possible functions the behaviours served were unique to each individual (see Table 8.1).

Table 8.1 *Challenging behaviour: a functional analysis of five cases*

	Behaviour (B)	Significant person variables/ unobservables	Functional meaning/purpose
Mary	Aggressive resistance	Private person	Maintenance of dignity and authority
	Abusive	Prone to anxiety	
	'Over-dressing'	A woman of standing and prestige	To assuage insecurities
Jack	Aggressive resistance	Apraxia	Frustration
	Violence		
Jane	Aggressive resistance	Perceptual disturbance	Fear reduction
	Toileting difficulty	Fear of worms	
Violet	Yelling	Poor vision	Communication of insecurity
Betty	Aggressive resistance	Enjoyed caring for others	Communication of insecurity
	Falls	Loved children	A need for occupation
	Hallucinations	Enjoyed housework	
	Noise making	Private, quiet and self-contained	
	Violence		
	Grabbing others	Poor eyesight	
	Interference with other residents	Perseveration	
		Apraxia	

Once a number of explanations have been generated using a methodology similar to creative brainstorming, those hypotheses that seem to offer the greatest explanatory power are tested by altering the environment. Samson & McDonnell (1990) describe how to use a functional analysis to guide intervention that meets the needs of a person with challenging behaviour:

1   Conduct a detailed analysis of a person, their history and needs. Involve all who know them. Collect information on remaining strengths, as these may be the foundations for future change. Identify the factors which predispose a person to be challenging as well as those features which finally trigger the behaviour. An essential part of the information is to determine the function of the behaviour for the person. If we do not understand why it is happening our interpretation is destined to be faulty.
2   Form hypotheses about why someone has behaved in the way they have in the past and what is maintaining their behaviour at present.
3   Draw up a formulation from the competing hypotheses that represents your 'best guess'. This may contain one, or a combination of the original hypotheses. The formulation should state how the present situation might be changed.

Conclusion

When all areas of information have been collected and the observations have yielded a wealth of situational data, it is the role of the staff to discuss the findings and identify the critical determinants. Only then can we move to the next stage, which is to intervene in order to meet the needs of a person.

Functional analysis is founded on accurate observation and considered information gathering. Otherwise it is little more than 'armchair theorising'. As a result, seeking an explanation can be a lengthy process. Unfortunately, time is not always on our side, and human resources do not always allow for a rigorous period of monitoring. It is also the case that 'silent' behaviours, for example incontinence, and those that are 'continuous' as distinct from discrete, for example confusion, nocturnal wandering, apathy or withdrawal, do not easily lend themselves to an ABC analysis. Yet we do not have to discard the methodology outright, for the approach imposes a structure on our thinking. It enables us to understand what may be triggering and maintaining a person's challenging behaviour, as well as guiding us to consider the role of the broader context and the significance of the behaviour for the person. Gibson *et al,* (1995) describe how careful observation of current behaviour and detailed life history information together helped reduce agitation and increased well-being in a man with probable Alzheimer's disease. Once this man was known again and the pattern of his restless behaviour was acknowledged, a once jovial man who had fallen silent and withdrawn into a private world again experienced 'relaxation and enjoyment'.

As we enter a new millennium, functional analysis is without doubt a formidable weapon to be employed in the pursuit of positive person-centred work. The conceptual and methodological expansion involved in its development provides an effective counter to the criticisms that behavioural analysis is an inadequate approach to understanding challenging behaviour.

CHAPTER 9
Resolution Therapy
....

A THEME OF THIS BOOK IS THAT dementia resonates meaning. Unfortunately, words and actions tend to conceal a dementing person's psychology. Yet, as was advocated earlier (p 66), an objective of person-centred work must be to decipher the communications and behaviour observed in dementia, to unearth the cryptic messages and acknowledge that the person is not lost but merely buried beneath the remnants of their cognitive powers. Such material is not readily accessible, but it is potentially recoverable.

The previous two chapters have described methodologies designed to provide us with insights into 'why they do what they do', approaches based upon observation, reasoning, inference and intuition. Could we not, as a complementary, if not alternative, approach, ask the people themselves what they are doing and how they are feeling, even though so many people believe there is little merit in talking to those with dementia? 'It is frequently thought that those who have dementia are unable to communicate appropriately, either with their carers or with each other, and that much of their conversation is doomed to be meaningless' (Frank, 1995). So are we able to make meaningful contact with a person with dementia? Is it possible to break through the barrier of linguistic pathology?

While not specific to challenging behaviour, resolution therapy (Goudie & Stokes, 1989; Stokes & Goudie, 1990) strives to achieve effective communication, thereby demonstrating that 'people with dementia have something to say and they do say it' (Frank, 1995). It can therefore provide valuable insights into the origins of demanding and disturbed behaviour. It requires a gentle touch, for we should never trample on a person's communications and impose our interpretation. But if we listen to their attempts to describe their subjective world, are alert to the possibility that speech contains metaphors of their experience and aware that behaviour may possess hidden messages, then our understanding deepens, for we are no longer merely hearing and responding to 'observable' signals, but instead are attempting to grasp the sense conveyed by their apparently meaningless conduct.

First introduced by Goudie & Stokes (1989), resolution therapy lies within the person-centred tradition of Rogerian humanistic psychology (Rogers, 1951). Through acceptance of the person and empathising with the motivations and emotions which lie behind the disintegrated verbal and behavioural expressions, we adopt what Stokes & Goudie (1990) called 'level 2 analysis'. In other words we move away from 'observables' (that is, words and actions – level 1 analysis) and reach behind the barrier of cognitive destruction that conceals and distorts so much of the person and gain access to the subjective world of need and feeling.

I have never forgotten an elderly woman who in the late beginnings of dementia would sit wringing her hands. When comforted, she would repeat over and over again, 'Fella like me'. What was she communicating? In accordance with Rogerian principles, gentle exploration and 'reflection of feelings' provided me with a probable explanation, a meaning that was confirmed when the person she was closest to was present. Only then would she be calm and her eyes brighten. This was not her husband, for she had been a widow for over 40 years, but her brother – that 'fella like me'.

The methodology has its limitations. We are not embarking upon a radical reinterpretation of human communication. Instead we are acknowledging that the articulations and actions of people with dementia are likely to mean something and, if we employ proven counselling qualities and skills that enable others to communicate more of themselves, then it is just possible that we might learn something from their fragmented and seemingly incomprehensible utterances. We are then better placed to work out what the meaning is and to acknowledge, rather than deny, the emotions, invariably painful, which are the natural accompaniments of the experience of dementia.

Resolution in Practice

Resolution Therapy is a one-to-one therapeutic approach to be conducted with sensitivity, patience and tolerance. It is not practised at certain times, in sessions or groups, but characterises the everyday interaction between all who come into contact with those with dementia. It entails paying attention to all attempts at communication. In care settings it is best practised by those in closest and most frequent contact with the person. Seen in this way, resolution therapy enhances the role of professional caregivers, for the importance attached to the motivations and phenomenological world of the individual requires a different kind of relationship between the person and carer from that which we most commonly observe in dementia care. It encourages carers to interact with a person with dementia in a meaningful way and challenges them to gain insights into a world that has historically been neglected. As Goudie & Stokes (1989) stated: 'Nurses are in daily contact and communication with dementing patients and, therefore, have an enormous therapeutic potential for this approach.'

It is at this face-to-face level where care is delivered that the quality of relationships is considered to have the greatest beneficial effect on well-being. Person-centred work is incompatible with interactions that are defined by their mechanical and perfunctory remoteness. It is the depth and quality of human relationships that demonstrates the value and worth we place on a person with dementia.

The focus of our communication is to understand *what* the person is trying to express through their apparently meaningless speech or behaviour. By reflecting on what is heard, seen and emotionally expressed, the 'therapist' attempts to understand the world from the point of view of the person with dementia. Tentative attempts are made to identify and acknowledge the feelings that might accompany the message. Their statements are not disputed, nor are they presented with reality. We endeavour to flow with their feelings.

It is essential to accept that we are not demanding explanations. Rather, we are attempting to understand what is happening and to acknowledge the feelings that are inextricably involved. In this way a person may feel enough at ease to share more of themselves and the reasons for their behaviour; the meaning of their actions will perhaps emerge as part of the 'unravelling process'.

The Core Personal Qualities

The publication in 1957 of a paper entitled 'The Necessary and Sufficient Conditions of Therapeutic Personality Change' (Rogers, 1957) outlined the three main attitudes, or 'ways of being', that help us communicate with people in distress. For 'perhaps more than anything else, Carl Rogers was a student of human communication' (Merry, 1995). Today, 'the evidence for the necessity, if not sufficiency, of the therapist conditions of accurate empathy, respect or warmth, and therapeutic genuineness is incontrovertible' (Patterson, 1984).

Resolution therapy is an invocation to use the core Rogerian counselling principles to communicate with people who have dementia. We are not talking about the use of techniques, but are instead addressing the domain of attitude, personal quality and interpersonal warmth: in other words, the quality of human relationships – a commitment to an authentic meeting of equals in which an individual with dementia is cared for and respected as a person, and where those who care see them as much more than a set of symptoms of a disease, residing 'in a body from which the former occupant has departed' (Morton, 1999). Only when we see beyond the illness and know we are working with a person like ourselves will there be motivation to empathise with that person's inner reality. Techniques and intellectual property can never be a substitute for these humanistic values.

Empathy

Empathy means being able to see the world through the eyes of someone else, stepping into their shoes as it were, and putting aside our own expectations and experiences as far as we are able. It is not the same as remembering how things were for us. It is what is referred to as entering another person's frame of reference, while holding onto a clear sense of our own identity.

At times of trouble there is likely to be somebody in your family or amongst your friends to whom you go to confide and share your worries.

They listen, are interested in what you say and how you feel, never judge and seem to understand as if they have also shared your experience, even though you know they have not. That depth of understanding is empathy, empathy that needs to be communicated to the person, for it is not of much use unless it is known that you understand. How we communicate 'your sensings of the person's world' (Rogers, 1980) will become clear as we consider the other 'core conditions' and skills necessary for person-centred communication.

Achieving empathy with people who have severe dementia is not without difficulty, however. We may find it easier to empathise with those who are at the beginning of the process of change, and know they are losing control and experiencing the loss of memory and knowing:

> Very difficult to concentrate. Memory is bad. Barbara gets exasperated with me and often I don't know why. There is a silent physical buzzing in my head. Is it depression or something worse …? A very disoriented day. Thoughts and actions seem to be slipping from my grasp – fog-like experience, slightly blurred. Have to concentrate in order to sort what I want to think – a kind of translucent cloud envelopes the words I am writing. Probably tiredness … Don't tell anyone!!! (The words of Malcolm, from *Malcolm and Barbara, A Love Story*, Granada Television, June 1999)

To enter the experience of those who have progressed beyond this and occupy a permanent world of not knowing, unable to attach meaning to what they see, is more difficult (Morton, 1999). The limitation of our own experience may place obstacles in our way, yet if we are determined to understand and prepared to check and adjust our understanding moment by moment, then as we become sensitive to the 'felt meanings' that flow from them, we become a confident companion in their inner world (Rogers, 1980).

Congruence
Congruence means we are *genuine* in our respect for the person with dementia. The image you present must match what is going on inside. Do not add to a person's puzzlement by presenting in one way but

saying something else. Congruence is contrary to adopting an objective, uninvolved or distant attitude (Merry, 1995). There can be no disguising feelings behind a professional façade. Any incongruence is likely to be picked up by the person and will undermine the therapeutic relationship (Morton, 1999), so you need to ask yourself, do you genuinely believe that we work with those who are our equals or is it lip service to fine aspirations?

Unconditional Positive Regard
Unconditional positive regard (or warmth or prizing) means we do not condemn or judge those with dementia. We prize the person no matter what they do: 'Accept your client without judgement' (Feil, 1992). Even though we might object to their challenging behaviour, this does not extend to condemning or being dismissive of them. We accept the person with dementia for who they are: a person struggling with life, yet doing their best, not someone to be regarded as a 'problem'.

These core 'ways of being' provide a non-threatening atmosphere. If we meet the person with dementia in a non-judgemental and understanding way, we hope that more complex layers of meaning and feeling will gradually emerge at the person's own pace and in his or her own way. It is the personal qualities we bring to the relationship that are most significant in determining whether the episode of communication will be successful, not our learning, 'cleverness' or special techniques. This does not mean that there are no skills involved, but these are seen as the means by which 'therapeutic workers' put their values and concern for others into practice, skills that pertain to good listening and clear communication (Merry, 1995).

The Skills of Resolution

'Patient attentive listening, retention and use of small details, empathetic responses to a person's expressed feeling ... help us to decode the symbolic non-verbal and fragmented communication used by many people with dementia' (Gibson *et al,* 1995). Our objectives are clear, but how does the process of resolution therapy unfold? Let us consider a communication with Terry.

The Setting Scene

Terry is leaving his home to enter respite care for a week. It is the first time during the course of his dementia that he has been apart from his wife. She is going away for a break with her daughter. She is exasperated with him. In many ways this is a trial period prior to a probable permanent placement.

He is standing, facing his son, looking bemused. Two members of staff from the residential home where he will be staying are present. There is an atmosphere of being rushed, for they have one other person to collect, and already they are behind schedule.

Received Message

Terry starts to call out, 'Where am I going? I am not going anywhere without my cat – no, no, no. Where's my cat?' He starts to call his cat's name. He is agitated and becomes resistive as his son attempts to hold his arm. Terry continues calling out the cat's name, yet his cat died several years ago. With 'level 1 analysis', his words demonstrate confusion (he is corrected, to no avail), but is this so? Using level 2 analysis, we enter Terry's frame of reference and determine whether his speech is an attempt at communication.

Pace

The communication cannot be rushed. The person, probably aged, affected not only by dementia but possibly by failing eyesight and poor hearing as well, needs time to express themselves. Pace is particularly important for achieving successful communication. We need to be in synchrony with the person's best pace. This can be achieved through monitoring and adjusting the speed of our communication, and learning to appreciate that pauses are not barren spells to be filled with our contribution, but a time during which the person is learning they are safe and attempting to articulate more about themselves.

These silences, even when measured in a few short seconds can be disarming, yet they are rarely inactive. The gift of silence is required so thoughts can be ordered and verbalised. So we allow time for responses to be formulated. Remember, it is the person we need to listen to, not ourselves. As a guide, it may be useful when a pause occurs to count to 10 slowly in your head before breaking the silence.

So beware haste. Unfortunately, for those in the life of Terry, time is of the essence. Their interaction is shallow. There is little regard for Terry's experience. They are concerned with the practical task of returning to the home with their residents. There is no malicious intent, but their relationship is subverted by the pressures of work. Hence they hear, but are not listening.

Focused Listening

Therapeutic listening can be difficult for it is not always easy to concentrate on what is being said. Think how often you have 'switched off' when somebody is so full of their own importance that all they do is talk about themselves. Perhaps you drifted off in a lecture? Perhaps you were only aware of having done so when your partner jolted you back to reality with the words, 'Have you heard a single word I've been saying?' Despite our best intentions, we may struggle to attend. This especially applies when we are listening to dementia speech. So 'to appreciate another person's frame of reference we must first learn to listen' (Morton, 1999).

Speech in dementia is not only characterised by paraphasia (that is, use of the wrong word order or the wrong word), neologisms (meaningless verbalisations) and circumlocution; content is also sparse, repetitious, disjointed and, at times, incomprehensible.

As an illustration, Frank (1995) records the following conversation between two people with dementia:

Laura: You see me in one place one time, and another place (( )) another time.
Stanley: Hm.
Laura: Anywhere it says hello [pause] (( )).
Stanley: [pause] (( )) goes, that's how it GOES.
Laura: Eh?
Stanley: How it goes, isn't it? [pause]
(( )) = not clearly intelligible speech.

Listening to such communications is demanding. Despite this dissolution of language, we have to be sensitive to the hidden messages and adjust to the observation that 'the language used by people with dementia is a metaphorical one' (Killick, 1994). We have to ask what words might represent (see p65) and then follow this previously concealed line of enquiry. It may not just be the words that are spoken which are important, the number of times they are said may also be significant. The repetition of particular words or phrases may reflect a key theme to be picked up.

We cannot afford to just listen. We must attend and listen with purpose. Good listening is always focused (Goodall *et al,* 1994). Yet this was not happening with Terry. The others heard him ask for his cat and immediately assumed he was confused. They did not listen and then address the possible meaning of his verbalisation: 'I need security. I need the security of my past when life was safe and predictable. I need to be soothed and comforted.'

Non-Verbal Signals
Our understanding of a person is not solely dependent on the words they use. While we listen to the messages and feelings beneath the words we can reach their complex inner world by also taking note of non-verbal clues.

Crimmens (1995) considers people with dementia are in a post-verbal stage. An infant is pre-verbal, yet we still bond and communicate. In no way is the absence of language an insuperable barrier to understanding. At times it is challenging, yet only occasionally are we defeated. However, even in adulthood, a time when we consider ourselves to be dependent on language to communicate, it is estimated that 'words constitute only 7 per cent of the information we pick up from someone in any one interaction' (ibid). The other 93 per cent is non-verbal; it is what we see and experience in terms of voice tone, intonation, facial expression, eye contact, hand movements, touch, body posture and physical distance. Words are just one component of the spectrum of communication. Sometimes the words say one thing but the non-verbals reveal another, suggesting that the person feels very differently. Respond to these non-verbal signs.

As language fails in dementia, it is clearly unwise to focus exclusively on verbal skills, for words are no longer the person's primary source of communication. So if we remain aware that we all express our thoughts and feelings in non-verbal ways, we have the key to developing the skills necessary to initiate and maintain meaningful contact with those with dementia.

Terry was bemused, agitated and unwelcoming of touch. Without doubt his non-verbal signals resonated his emotional state of distress and confirmed the concealed need for reassurance – reassurance that was not forthcoming. He was simply told his cat was dead!

Active Listening

The objective of resolution therapy is for the person to disclose more of themselves. We need to listen with empathy, but we must also communicate that we are listening. Too often others present as uninterested when faced with the 'ramblings' of a dementing person. They look away, respond inappropriately and make cursory comments. You can tell they are thinking 'I have better things to do than stand here ...' How did you feel when you knew that you did not have the undivided attention of the person you were talking to? Embarrassed, awkward, angry, insignificant? Were you encouraged to talk more? Or did you feel there was no point continuing, for they were not really listening? It can be humiliating talking to someone whose mind appears to be elsewhere, or who appears indifferent to what you have to say. We need to know somebody is listening. If you do not believe this is so, try talking to another person sitting back to back, having asked the listener to say as little as possible. You will soon be wishing to know whether they are still listening and how they feel about what you are saying. It is no different for those with dementia. Despite deteriorating cognitive faculties, they remain intuitive and sensitive to mood. People with dementia can be superb barometers of the interpersonal climate. So does the prevailing culture set the scene for the development of communication, or does it tend to 'close down' attempts to communicate because we show we are not listening?

Goodall *et al* (1994) detail the interpersonal characteristics we can use to engage someone's attention and then maintain that communication.

Posture If sitting, a relaxed, open posture, with arms and legs uncrossed will help the other person feel relaxed as well. You will find it easier to concentrate on the person if you face them, perhaps leaning slightly forward, and they are more likely then to feel that you are focusing on them. Do not however present as intimidating by violating their personal space and leaning over them.

Eye contact When they look at you, make eye contact. This is reassurance that you are listening attentively and may encourage them to talk further. If they wish to hand the conversation to you, they will continue to look at you until you pick it up. Too much eye contact may appear confrontational; too little will give the impression that we are either not interested or uncertain of ourselves.

Facial expression The capacity to smile is a basic social signal that generates warmth and encourages human contact. If we smile, they smile. It is a reassuring, calming sign (Burgener *et al*, 1992).

Voice tone Aim for a gentle tone to reassure and so encourage them to say more. Do not, however, talk so gently that they cannot hear what you say. You may use a puzzled tone to encourage them to reflect on what they have said.

Gesture Gestures help to punctuate a conversation. When it is hard to convey in words your feeling for what the person is saying, a gesture may be the most adequate response you can make.

Touch Touch can provide stability in the midst of muddle, frustration and emotional chaos. Touch can say 'I am with you, I am listening,' when words are inadequate. At the same time, we must recognise that some people feel uncomfortable with touch. Thus the appropriateness of physical contact must always be monitored at this time, with this person. Do they tense when you touch them, or pull away?

When using touch, do so with confidence, rather than apologetically.

Uhms and nods Sounds of acknowledgement are useful for conveying that you are listening and encouraging the person to continue.

Reflective Listening
We are attempting to gain access to the person's subjective experience and to find out what their words mean, what they know themselves to be doing and how they are feeling. Yet it is not for us to demand explanations. In fact, it is not for us to say much at all. What we do say, however, is important in showing that we are listening, we understand

and we want them to say more. Our words are simply the vehicle to enable us to find out more about the person.

Particularly important is reflecting back to the person. By repeating and clarifying what they have said, we do not lead but provide a series of stepping stones enabling the person to step onto the next level of disclosure. There are various ways we can do this:

- repeating a key word,
- repeating a short phrase the person has used,
- paraphrasing the main theme of what they have just been saying,
- reflecting on what the person is feeling,
- reflecting on what the person has done or is doing.

It is important to recognise that what you reflect to the person is likely to influence the subsequent course of the conversation.

We do not simply reflect their words or our construction of their words, we respond to their perceptions of themselves and the world around them, and how they are expressing themselves emotionally. In this sense we talk of 'reflection of feelings'. However, reflecting listening is more complex than making simple reflections:

> I am trying to determine whether my understanding of the client's inner world is correct – whether I am seeing it as he or she is experiencing it at this moment. Each response of mine contains the unspoken question, 'Is this the way it is for you?' Am I catching just the colour and texture and flavour of the personal meaning you are experiencing right now? (Rogers, 1986)

If the answer is 'no', we need to bring our thinking in to line with theirs. All attempts to reflect and acknowledge feelings experienced by the person with dementia must be tentative until confirmation is received. Flexibility of response and monitoring reaction to our acknowledgements are cornerstones of resolution therapy (Stokes & Goudie, 1990).

Van Werde & Morton (1999) believe that reflective listening can help family carers to cope. A son used 'contact reflections' to keep a conversation going with his mother by constantly reflecting concrete reality. (For example, when she stumbled over the words 'hot ... heat (( )) ho...', he reflected, 'It is warm'. She then gestured she was thirsty.) His 'conversation' with her became bearable and gave him a feeling that his mother felt herself to be understood.

With Terry, on hearing him shout out for his cat, those around him may have reflected:

'You seem troubled, Terry?'
'Maybe you are feeling a bit nervous about coming to Windsor Lodge? Most people do when they visit us for the first time.'
'Your cat is important to you?'
'You feel bad now.'

Whether Terry replies and expands on his vocalisations depends on him. We cannot force people to engage with us. If Terry is either unable or unwilling to do so he will not communicate. Having presented him with a sensitive interpersonal context we can do little more. It is important to realise that 'sometimes with the best will in the world the person does not want to engage with you right now, and that is a choice that person is making and not a bad reflection on you' (Crimmens, 1995).

The challenge of establishing 'psychological contact' can be difficult, yet through the practice of Pre-therapy with people with psychosis and learning difficulties Prouty (1994) offers us hope. Pre-therapy is conceived as a means of facilitating psychological contact as a 'pre-condition' of 'therapy'. Van Werde & Morton (2000), in a fine exposition of the approach describe fundamental skills such as 'Word-for-Word Reflections' to initiate contact. They assert that the aim of Pre-therapy 'is to open up areas of mental health that have remained largely neglected by person-centred theorists and practitioners'.

Questions
A barrage of questions is not required. It is even the case that the careful use of non-verbal skills and reflection may result in very few questions being asked. We must 'just let them talk'.

If questions are asked, try to avoid open-ended questions (Enderby, 1990). Open questions are those that cannot be answered in one word and as a result can encourage a person to give more information. As a result, they are favoured by therapists. However, in dementia such questioning can be too complex in terms of reasoning and linguistics. It is better to ask closed questions which can often be answered with a 'yes' or 'no', or by a short phrase. These questions help to clarify events and fill in details which may be crucial to our understanding of a situation. For a person who is struggling to communicate, such questions may encourage them to at least contribute a one word answer.

As with reflective responses, questions can pick up on feelings, thoughts, actions or meaning (Goodall *et al*, 1994). Do not ask multiple questions as these can be bewildering. Questioning should be straightforward, concise and concrete, for example:

'Terry, are you worried?'
'Do you know where we're going?'
'Do you know who I am, Terry?'
'Are you angry with us?'

General Guidelines for Communication

Enderby (1990) provides useful guidance for promoting successful communication:

- Reduce background noise that can be a source of distraction and may interfere with hearing and comprehension.
- Raise the voice slightly at the beginning to gain their attention.
- Use short sentences, with simple grammatical structures.
- If comprehension is poor, use different ways of saying the same thing, so the person receives the message in two or three different ways.
- Your words should be unambiguous.
- Encourage the person with dementia to communicate in whatever way is appropriate.
- Encourage them to gesture.

If these guidelines are followed, good communication is facilitated and resolution therapy commences: a move toward appreciating and attempting to understand the meanings and feelings that lie behind the words and actions observed in dementia; a sense which is discernible as more of their subjective experience is disclosed; an understanding that is guided by a knowledge of the person and an appreciation of our shared humanity. Our dialogue demonstrates that we are no longer responding to errors and mistaken beliefs. It is their phenomenology which is of importance. Resolution therapy is designed to help us make contact with that person who can no longer communicate as they once did, yet through their often unintelligible behaviour is continuing to demonstrate their 'personhood'.

CHAPTER 10

Resolution: Needs to be Met, not Problems to be Managed

THE NEW CULTURE OF DEMENTIA CARE recognises the human value and worth of a person. Through observation, empathy and becoming a better listener we endeavour to understand the needs and struggles of the person with dementia. However, despite our acceptance of the person, the language of engagement still continues to be in terms of 'problem behaviours', a language that encourages a call to the doctor for help and is a step away from the introduction of measures to 'control' and 'manage'. Our concern has become the problem, not the person. How can we reframe so-called 'problem behaviours' so that we do not lose sight of person-centred values?

Needs or Problems?

So much challenging behaviour is in the realm of need, even if it is simply the need to have agency and be oneself (that is, comfortable behaviours). Challenging actions not to be just understood and tolerated, but if necessary and possible to be resolved. However, our efforts to see such behaviour as a real challenge to all involved to find a way forward, rather than a problem residing in the person (Woods, 1995) can be compromised if we move away from overt acknowledgements of need and instead assume that the meanings and motivations behind behaviour are accepted by all. To ensure that this does not happen, we are required to communicate the challenge of their behaviour by 'operationalising' the concept of need.

Behavioural Deficits

The Language of Need and Individual Goal Planning
People with dementia present us with two types of challenge, behavioural deficits and behavioural excesses. Deficits are actions they no longer perform but we wish they did (known as acts of omission). In other words, we observe dependency. They are dependent inasmuch as they:

wet themselves	cannot take care of their appearance
withdraw from others	cannot pursue purposeful activity
cannot dress	cannot feed themselves
neglect their personal hygiene	
cannot take responsibility for their financial affairs	
mislay household items	

Operational definitions of these behavioural deficits enable us to know exactly what is being communicated by these statements (see Chapter 2), yet the language remains negative. For that is what problems are, a negative appraisal of a person's actions. Needs are problems restated in positive terms. We move on from the operational definition by making a clear statement of need. For example, 'Mr Brady is withdrawn' might be rephrased as 'Mr Brady needs companionship'. The need domain is sociability. We have stated what the person needs or needs to do, rather than dwelling on the problem as a negative issue and just describing what happens. Similarly, we might say, 'Mrs Parlour needs to toilet appropriately', having initially described her behaviour as 'Mrs Parlour keeps urinating on the floor by her chair'. Or 'Mrs Hughes needs to remember where she puts her keys,' rather than 'Mrs Hughes mislays her personal possessions'.

Although stating problems as needs in positive terms like this may seem long-winded, as if we are playing with words, focusing on the person this way gives a sense of direction and indicates what can be achieved, rather than seeing them as a collection of problems which carers have to cope with (Goudie, 1990). It is said that communicating a person's difficulties in the language of need places us on the road facing in the right direction, looking towards goals to be set, potential to be released and the expectation that change will occur. We have progressed from a lifeless statement of fact to a working statement of intent (Perrin, 1996). These aspirations are contrary to the institutionalised objective of disempowerment that dominated the old culture of dementia care. Instead, we wish them to utilise the remaining abilities of those with dementia and to receive assistance to help them complete actions they have initiated. The goal is assisted independence.

The next step is to enquire why the need is unmet. What is it about that person and/or their circumstances which prevents them from fulfilling their need? Obtaining the answer to this question can be helped by understanding that many self-care behaviours are the outcome of negotiating an intricate chain of actions that commences with the recognition of need. Elements of the chain are not in reality separate and independent atoms of behaviour but are interrelated skills and actions. The chain can break down at any point because of disease, disability, demotivation, emotional disorder, environmental factors or a mixture of all these.

Table 10.1 demonstrates the chain of behaviour that results in appropriate toileting. We can see that the points where the chain could snap correspond to the taxonomy of possible explanations for a toileting difficulty (summarised in Table 10.2). Only failure at the beginning of the chain is considered evidence of incontinence. The breakdown of the chain at other points follows an awareness of need, but the result is still dysfunctional, inappropriate behaviour.

However, just because the chain of adaptive behaviour snaps (and we could be now considering the failure to dress, shave, prepare food or any other self-care behaviour), we do not move in and disempower the person by taking over, submerging them in care and creating excess disabilities (Brody et al, 1971). Instead, we identify where the person has difficulty and embark upon an individualised plan of action. In the case of Mrs S (pp52–3) it was not for her to change, but for the environment to be adapted so it corresponded with her personal need for hygiene.

If, however, the dysfunctional behaviour can be addressed through change within the person, goal planning is the recommended option

Table 10.1 *The essential pathway to successful toileting*

1 Recognising the need to urinate and postponing within limits, the act of micturition (failure = incontinence).

2 Being motivated to use the toilet.

3 Possessing the physical strength and steadiness to stand.

4 Possessing the mobility, stamina and confidence to cover the distance to the toilet and overcome any obstacles along the way (for example, floor surfaces, stairs, outstretched legs of others).

5 Maintaining goal-oriented behaviour.

6 Being able to locate the toilet (or acceptable alternative).

7 Perceiving and experiencing the toilet as accessible, safe, hygienic and private.

8 Possessing the dexterity and co-ordination to adjust clothing.

9 Initiating the act of micturition.

Table 10.2 *Toileting difficulties: seeking understanding (a summary)*

Incontinence	localised physical abnormality (eg, urinary tract infection, enlargement of the prostate gland, constipation) cortical atrophy nocturnal enuresis
Neurogenesis	apraxia, aphasia, agnosia, memory loss
Sensory handicap	
Physical disability	mobility and dexterity
Medication effects	sedatives, anti-depressants, diuretics
Mood	
Built environment	distance, obstacles, safety
Social environment	attitudes and actions of others
Psychological factors	personality, habit, life experience, motivation

(Barrowclough & Fleming, 1986). Goal planning is a structured approach that draws upon a person's remaining strengths (that is, what they can do, and like to do, and who will be willing to help them), in order to help and motivate them towards tackling their difficulties and meeting their needs. For example, an anxious, withdrawn man who has retained the ability to make eye contact may benefit enormously from this non-verbal communication for it may go some way to meet his need to belong and feel secure. Yet carers often need to be helped to see strengths in people. As Perrin (1996) remarks, it is easy 'to see weakness (she can't walk far) rather than strength (she can still walk from her bedroom to the dining room)'.

Goudie (1990) describes how realistic goal plans are devised (realistic in terms of the person's residual abilities and what the care setting can realistically offer) and how these address in a positive way key questions such as what the person will do, who they will do it with, how they will do it and when they will do it. We accept that, for many people, goals will be limited in ambition, but the drive is always to help a person maximise their potential wherever possible. For example, if a person is no longer aware or motivated to use the toilet our intervention may take the form of building on the strengths that remain and introduce an individualised approach to promote toileting abilities and 'support autonomy', such as a Daytime Habit Retraining programme (Box 10.1), patterned urge response toileting (PURT) (Colling *et al*, 1992). Goudie *et al* (1990) identify ways that carers can help encourage and maintain skills in daily living activities, while Holden (1990b; 1995) provides practical and creative suggestions to help rehabilitate those whose dependency is the result of neuropsychological deficits such as apraxia, perseveration and agnosia. Perrin (1996) uses case studies to illustrate specific relearning methods, such as backward chaining (see Box 10.2). In all instances, the language of the new culture of care is evident: potential, rehabilitation, creativity and resolution. These are the guiding principles of our work.

Box 10.1 Daytime habit retraining

When a person's pattern of micturition guides the toileting programme, it is known as habit retraining. As inflexible toileting procedures should not be imposed upon people in care who reveal predictable toileting needs, this approach has much to recommend it. It can be an effective strategy to employ in those cases where a toileting difficulty arises because of, for example, demotivation or disability, which prevent independent toileting ever being a realistic goal.

The objective is to remind the person to void at intervals which will anticipate incidents of wetting in order to produce an acceptable toileting rhythm.

In the beginning, as with patterned urge response toileting (PURT), a person is initially checked at fixed intervals, say every two hours, to establish whether they are wet or dry. They are then prompted and assisted to use the toilet. The outcome of this intervention is recorded on a Habit Retraining Assessment Chart, which can take the form of the example below:

Habit Retraining Assessment Chart

TIME	am							pm							
Day	Date	8.00	9.00	10.00	11.00	12.00	1.00	2.00	3.00	4.00	5.00	6.00	7.00	8.00	9.00
		C T	C T	C T	C T	C T	C T	C T	C T	C T	C T	C T	C T	C T	C T

KEY	State of resident (C)	Result of toileting (T)
C = Check	D = Dry	Passed urine = Blue dot
T = Toilet use	W = Wet	Not passed urine = Red dot
		Refused = oblique line (/)

Information is recorded on whether a person was found wet and whether the prompt to use the toilet resulted in the passing of urine or not. It is desirable to keep the number of occasions when voiding does not occur to a minimum and thus there is a need to identify those visits to the toilet which were unnecessary.

If a pattern of micturition is revealed over a number of days (at least three), then the person is suitable for habit retraining. At those times when the person was found to be consistently wet, adjustments are made to the schedule to allow them to be accompanied to the toilet before voiding occurs. Similarly, visits to the toilet may be discontinued if a person has regularly failed to void when taken to the toilet. In this way the programme is amended according to the person's needs.

For example, the following results may be obtained:

	8.00 am	10.00 am	12.00 noon	2.00 pm	4.00 pm	6.00 pm	8.00 pm
Check	Wet	Wet	Dry	Dry	Wet	Wet	Dry
Toilet use	Yes	No	Yes	No	No	Yes	Yes

Observation has revealed episodes of wetting at 8.00 am, 10.00 am, 4.00 pm and 6.00 pm, and non-usage of the toilet at 10.00 am, 2.00 pm and 4.00 pm.

To pre-empt inappropriate urinating, the schedule is adjusted so that toilet prompts take place a half hour earlier than the original check times when the person was discovered wet. In addition, those checks where the person was found to be dry and the prompt to use the toilet did *not* result in the passing of urine are now discontinued.

The resulting schedule of toilet prompts, is as follows: 7.30 am, 9.30 am, 12.00 noon, 3.30 pm, 5.30 pm and 8.00 pm.

As you can see the number of toilet visits has been reduced to six from the original seven, so not only does this procedure benefit the person, who is saved the indignity of unnecessary toileting, it also allows for a more efficient use of caregiver time.

The final stage in habit retraining is to extend the intervals between prompts by 15 minutes until three-hourly intervals are established throughout the day. Following a successful outcome to this stage, prompted toileting will have been markedly reduced.

As a result of adjusting and extending the time between toileting prompts so that voiding is postponed for as long as possible, a new pattern of predictable micturition is established which enables the person with dementia to remain dry, as well as avoiding fruitless journeys to the toilet.

Box 10.2 Backward chaining: on the path to 'rementia', a toileting difficulty

This method of relearning starts at the end of the sequence of toileting behaviours. We establish the final step first and only then go on to the preceding link in the chain. For example, you can concentrate initially on the person's ability to rearrange clothing after toilet use. Once practice in this dressing skill has established the behaviour, you then focus on the act of voiding while at the toilet. Eventually, you direct your intervention towards the 'approach' behaviours, such as finding the way to the toilet, getting up and walking to the toilet, and ultimately making the decision to go to the toilet when necessary. Each component part of the chain of toileting skills can be relearned in this way. Learning is encouraged by the use of social reinforcers (these may be verbal, as in a remark of gentle praise, or physical, as with a squeeze of the hand).

The advantage of backward chaining is that the completion of the chain possesses the reward of fulfilment. Concentrating on the skills closest to completion will motivate relearning. Once these have been acquired, preceding steps can be learned with the knowledge that the chain can be completed. This again serves to encourage the goal of 'rementia'.

Multi-Modal Intervention: The Objective is Prevention

A multi-modal approach to intervention is a preventive methodology that is integrated within the culture of care. It is a global environmental response to the challenge of dependency that trawls the known causes of a specific dependent behaviour and attempts to avoid, compensate or accommodate the reasons for the unmet need.

The multi-modal approach lends itself to those self-care needs that can be understood as involving a number of component steps that require adequate environmental conditions for the chain to be completed. Stokes (1990c; 1995c) described how the approach has shown itself to be a successful therapeutic strategy when working with the challenge of 'toileting difficulty', helping many people to avoid the degrading experience of being found wet or soiled.

The adoption of multi-modal principles does not meet the needs of all people, nor is it applicable to all behavioural deficits. At these times individualised goal planning may be the most effective means of reducing dependency, by motivating and helping people to do as much for themselves as possible, for as long as possible.

Behavioural Excesses

Framing Challenging Behaviours as Needs
Behavioural excesses are the principal concern of this book. These acts of commission are unwanted, unwelcome, superficially demonstrate the person 'is lost' and give rise to desperation among family carers as they protest that they cannot cope with what their relative has started to do.

Again we must move away from negative expressions to positive restatement of need, but how is this to be achieved? It is straightforward when working with dependency: we simply turn the negative into a positive. So 'she can't dress' becomes 'she needs to dress'; 'he won't get up' is rephrased as 'he needs to get out of bed', but how do we restate challenging behavioural excesses?

- Wandering – needs to walk further!
- Violence – needs to hit harder!
- Noise making – needs to shout louder!

Such 'positive' statements are not tenable. We cannot say 'needs to stop …' as this represents *our* need for peace and quiet. So does this imply that when we face behaviours that challenge our capacity to cope we are unable to employ the language of need, and must instead continue to envisage challenging behaviour in terms of 'problems', problems that can be legitimised by reference to symptoms of a disease with the attendant risk of resurrecting the primacy of the medical model? Thus, a care manager can identify with the needs of a stressed carer yet only sees the problem, no symptom of 'wandering'. The outcome is that the need of the carer for rest and peace of mind is met, the symptom is 'managed' by entry to respite care. With our commitment to *a person* with dementia it is hoped that unthinking service responses are less likely, yet without a clear statement of need we increase the likelihood of such actions occurring.

To restate an act of commission in the positive language of need, we do not rephrase the challenging behaviour (as we do with deficits in performance). Instead, having first determined the probable reason for the behavioural excess, we couch the explanation in positive terms and, as we have demonstrated time and time again, the explanation is not 'they have dementia'. For, if this remains our attitude, it is impossible to frame that in terms of a need. If a neurogenic cause is probable then we need to be specific (for example, frontal lobe syndrome, apraxia, Klüver-Bucy syndrome) and then consider the prospect of neuropsychological rehabilitation (see, for example, Holden, 1995; Moniz-Cook *et al*, 1999).

How we progress from the negative framework of challenging behaviours to a statement of need, and how this may be facilitated by pinpointing behavioural characteristics, is shown in Table 10.3.

The progression of our methodology of resolution is evident. We cannot resolve challenging behaviour, we can only resolve the *reasons* for such behaviour. Explanations are now expressed in terms of need. Even when the nature of need cannot be determined we continue to acknowledge the motivation, for example, an explanation for 'repetitive questioning' is a 'forlorn attempt to communicate need'; for 'noise making' we propose 'needs to be met'; 'wandering' may only be 'apparently aimless'.

Resolution

'Resolution therapy is ultimately concerned with finding ways to help the person meet their needs and cope with their feelings. These may include verbal and non-verbal acknowledgements as well as modifications to the environment and carer–dependant relationships' (Stokes & Goudie, 1990).

I am often asked, 'What can be done?', yet without knowledge of the client and their worlds, both subjective and external, I can offer little other than general advice and suggestions. For example, there are good practice guidelines to encourage sleep, thereby reducing the prospect of 'nocturnal disturbance' (see Morgan & Gledhill, 1991; Wolfe & Herzberg, 1996). Bright light therapy has been shown to be effective in reducing 'sundowning', although not in all cases (Satlin *et al*, 1991; Lovell *et al*,

Table 10.3 *Challenging behaviours: possible explanations and the expression of need*

Behaviour	Behavioural characteristic	Possible explanation	Need
Wandering	pottering with purpose	boredom	to be occupied
Wandering	trailing and tracking	separation anxiety	to be secure
Wandering	pacing	anxiety and agitation	to be calm
Noise making	groaning	pain	to be pain free
Toileting difficulty*	using an inappropriate receptacle	(i) disorientation (ii) agnosia	(i) to find their way (ii) to recognise
Aggression	physical assault	defensive behaviour	to be informed
Hoarding		insecurity	to be secure
Noise-making	yelling	environmental discomfort	to be comfortable
Repetitive questioning		hard of hearing	to hear
Placing inedible objects in the mouth		curiosity	to know
Repetitive questioning		loneliness	to have companionship

Note: *an act of both omission and commission.

1995). Then there is guidance on activity programming, so helping to prevent boredom-induced challenges (for example, pottering with purpose, noise making). These are described in Box 10.3.

Box 10.3 Guidelines for activity and stimulation in dementia care
The need for occupation can be met in several ways.

- For those who are more able, activities that are culture-appropriate, age-relevant and, most significantly, address their individual pleasures and interests are of value, as are activities that help to maintain lifestyle skills. These are more to do with daily living than pastimes and may serve to promote self-respect and competence (see Briscoe, 1990).
- For those who do not wish to be active they can enjoy the pleasures of passive stimulation: a pleasant view, a sunny place, or 'smelling the products of someone else's baking session or having the cat on their lap' (Briscoe, 1990).
- The losses experienced by people with advanced dementia lead to many being left in chairs dozing or abandoned to pace corridors, with carers arguing that nothing can be done as they are beyond occupation. Yet ability is not always relevant. We simply need to broaden our understanding of occupational need and appreciate the benefits of non-cognitive stimulation. Perrin (1995) argues that we need to engage in activities that are neither skills-based nor dependent upon outcome for value, but instead appeal to the senses 'and the emotions which can appreciate them'. We can explore a person's sensory avenues through the use of natural sounds, music and movement (Hook, 1998), aromatherapy (West & Brockman, 1994) and evocative smells; tactile approaches such a massage; and the visual display of changing colours and moving patterns of scenes or abstract shapes (Dowling *et al*, 1997). The attraction of multi-sensory experience has led to 'Snoezelen rooms' appearing in dementia care settings, but while sensory stimulation is of demonstrable benefit, the unfamiliar Snoezelen environment is of questionable utility.
- For those who are confined to their bed or chair, Briscoe (1990) highlights the benefits of fabric textures and scented pillows.

In essence, however, the person-centred model of dementia, is incompatible with both generalised interventions and prescribed practice. We cannot prescribe procedures to resolve a person's difficulties in the same way as medication is administered, and it is the continuing dominance of thinking associated with the medical model that encourages many to wish for 'off-the-shelf' solutions. Resolution is focused on the individual and their needs; is specific to them and their circumstances; and our solutions may even be contrary to accepted practice – remember our intervention with Mrs O (p78). In certain instances empathic acknowledgement of feelings may be sufficient to achieve well-being (as may have been the case with Terry, p160). On other occasions the primary drive of resolution is to introduce changes to the psychosocial milieu and physical environment so that needs are no longer denied or frustrated. Once we have worked out the nature of, and motivation for, their actions we act to improve the situation, rather than merely acknowledging the behaviour and accompanying feelings.

Case Studies of Resolution
To provide insights into the person-centred approach to challenging behaviour we have informed the process through a number of case studies, illustrations that have demonstrated how resolution was achieved through the meeting of need. We have considered the experiences of Patrick (p51), Mrs S (p52), Mrs O (p78), Ron (p104) and Ian (p136) and how their needs have been acknowledged and met. To further our appreciation of how resolution is achieved, let us complete the story of Mrs D.

As we saw earlier (p104), Mrs D had a dread of the 'colour purple', in her faith a colour associated with death and mourning. At night, her room made her so fearful she was psychologically comfortable only when elsewhere. Her need to feel secure was met when she changed places with another resident and moved into a room that was colour co-ordinated light and dark green. From the first night, she slept soundly with no sign of distress. Once the motivation for her disturbed night-time behaviour was understood, resolution was straightforward. Yet the outcome could have been very different.

Prior to the identification of the probable origins of her behaviour, Mrs D was deemed 'unmanageable'. I cannot exaggerate the extent to which she disturbed the unit at night: so much so that following the failure of sedation, a transfer to a continuing care ward at the local psychiatric hospital had been arranged. However, the day before she was due to leave the home, the man with whom she was exchanging placements developed a chest infection. The transfer was suspended until he was restored to health. It was during this period that the nature of Mrs D's distress was clarified and the cause identified. Yet, if that gentleman had not fallen ill, Mrs D would already have been residing on a long-stay ward. Known to be disruptive at night – noisy, aggressive, a wanderer – she would have been given a major tranquilliser with sedative properties and condemned to live her final months on a run-down 'Nightingale' ward, a tragic consequence of staff failing to reach behind the barrier. In Mrs D's case, her violence was without doubt the voice of the unheard.

In similar vein, Moniz-Cook & Gill (1996) looked at examples of superstitious behaviour that may come to the fore during times of uncertainty and help our 'understanding of fearful, odd or "difficult" behaviour'. Consequently, in biographical history taking, religious, spiritual and superstitious beliefs should be part of individual care planning. There is a burgeoning literature on 'meeting spiritual needs' (for example, Froggatt, 1994; Barnett, 1995; Kitwood *et al*, 1995; Moffitt, 1996; Goodall, 1997). If formal faith is identified then access to collective worship can also provide a sense of belonging, the opportunity to express feelings and the security of a familiar ritual.

Most of the case studies reported so far have benefited from the methodologies of resolution therapy and creative brainstorming, at times informed by the structure imposed on our understanding by behavioural analysis. However, we conclude this chapter on resolution by looking in detail at interventions that were the outcome of (eco)behavioural and functional analysis. The language may be different, but the objectives are the same. While aspects of the methodology are shared with companion techniques (for example, gaining a knowledge of the person), the overall approach is distinguished by a period of formal observation and empirical rigour.

We left the story of Mr G (p150) at the point where behavioural analysis had demonstrated that his violent conduct was related to the intimate act of toileting him. Functional analysis revealed the 'person variables' that potentiated the behaviour – environment relationship. He had been a school teacher, a man used to respect, a person accustomed to being in charge. He was proud, stubborn, yet shy; a reserved man, but well-meaning and considerate of others. He did not enjoy company, and so it was unsurprising that his passion was gardening.

How were we to reconcile Mr G's need to be assisted to the toilet, with his need to ward off the invasive and threatening actions of others? Already staff were talking about incontinence pads and the benefits of using a catheter. The solution was the small garden where residents were able to walk safely.

As there did not appear to be a pattern to his episodes of wetting, a rigid toileting programme was introduced. Every two hours, Mr G was approached, yet he was never requested to use the toilet. Instead, staff worked in harmony with what they knew of his life history. Acknowledging his position as a teacher, they placed him in a position of authority and appealed to his well-meaning nature by seeking his advice with regard to whether the roses required pruning, the seedlings repotting, the greenfly infestation treating, or the lawn mowing. In other words, we blended an appreciation of his status with his enthusiasm for gardening.

The transformation was remarkable. Mr G would rise from his chair and offer his arm. He would be assisted along the corridor toward the garden, passing the two toilets for the unit. If he was accompanied by a male member of staff, the latter would say, 'I'm nipping in before we go outside, are you coming as well?' This would have been a customary practice for an enthusiastic gardener of his generation who might be outside for hours and would not wish to walk through the house with muddy boots in order to go upstairs to the toilet. If he was being accompanied by a woman, she would say, 'I've just been to the toilet. Do you wish to go? We could be outside for some time'. On nearly all occasions he would, at this point, toilet independently.

Mr G would then walk into the garden and be engaged in conversation. His manner was 'alive'. The content of his speech was largely unintelligible, but he was clearly relishing the experience. He was again the man he had once been. Staff would stay with him for a few minutes and then accompany him back into the home or he would stay outside until he wished to return. In winter the greenhouse was the salvation – not for Mr G, who would go outside in any weather, but for the staff who did not share his disregard for inclement weather!

In the beginning staff were sceptical: it would not work because:

- they did not believe in him as a person with a unique psychology and feelings,
- he would not agree to use the toilet,
- any suggestion to toilet would be met with aggressive resistance,
- he would remember the previous contrived episode and refuse to co-operate next time.

The approach, now empathic and sensitive, was successful. His old self was restored, and as for remembering the earlier approaches, how could he? Mr G was unable to remember for more than moments, let alone what had transpired two hours before.

During the two-week baseline period, 47 violent incidents had been recorded, in the 14 days that followed intervention, just six episodes of violence were observed, a demonstrable success that exercised a dramatic effect on staff perceptions. Mr G was no longer an 'objectified' individual degraded by dementia, but a man worthy of respect, with needs beyond the realms of physical care. Yet all we had done was to implement a basic toileting programme, but one informed by functional analysis. The outcome was a creative intervention.

Adopting a different behavioural approach to the challenge of inappropriate urinating, Bird *et al* (1995) worked with a man who urinated in the corners of rooms as a result of disorientation. His need was to find the way. Despite severe dementia, Max was taught to associate a large coloured sign with the location of the toilet. As a result, incidents of inappropriate voiding that had been occurring four or five times each day ceased.

Bird *et al* (ibid) make a modest claim for their intervention, inasmuch as they assert that the use of cued recall 'will be effective with some patients, with some problems, some of the time' (we will return to this methodology in the next chapter).

The previously mentioned study by Moniz-Cook *et al* (1999) explored the effects of individualised care plans following functional analysis (see Table 8.1). Single case experimental design was used to test empirically the hypotheses and associated interventions. Information was collected over a number of consecutive days during which time a baseline was determined and then the intervention was applied, withdrawn and applied again. Any improvement in performance could then be attributed to the intervention. The case profiles demonstrate the degree of therapeutic success achieved.

Mary 74 years old   Diagnosis: probable Alzheimer's disease

Challenging behaviour
1 Aggressive resistance during assistance with self-care.
2 Overdressing; that is, she wore all the clothes in her wardrobe, as well as clothes taken from other residents.

Formulation
1 Need for respect.
2 A means of coping with anxiety, for in her past she would go shopping for clothes or dress well in order to reassure herself.

Resolution
1 Staff were encouraged to converse with her about her significant life achievements, as well as to offer her a bath first, serve her first at mealtimes and to engage her first during social therapy groups.
2 Staff provided reassurance when she was anxious ('holding'). They encouraged competing adaptive behaviour by discussing her choice of clothing and jewellery when assisting with dressing.

Outcome
At three-month follow up, staff reported no aggressive resistance during bathing or mealtimes and a marked reduction in the frequency of overdressing.

Jack 80 years old   Diagnosis: probable vascular dementia

Challenging behaviour
Physical aggression during self-care tasks, especially when bathing.

Formulation
Neuropsychological examination revealed an apraxia which resulted

in his being unable to carry out activities when his movements were under voluntary control.

Resolution

Staff spoke to Jack about his hobbies and wartime experiences as they walked to the bathroom. Similar conversation-based distractors aimed at promoting automatic behaviour were employed during dressing and mealtimes.

Outcome

At three-month follow-up, on 9 out of 12 of occasions Jack bathed without difficulty.

Jane 79 years old Diagnosis: probable mixed Alzheimer's disease and vascular dementia

Challenging behaviour

Refusal to use the toilet as it 'was crawling with worms'. Would not accept a commode or incontinence pads.

Formulation

Perceptual disturbance led her to misperceive the black and white floor tiles in the toilet cubicle as being worms.

Resolution

The floor of the toilet cubicles was painted dark red.

Outcome

Independent use of the toilet.

Violet 88 years old Diagnosis: Dementia of unknown origin

Challenging behaviour

Yelling. Her screams were worst at times of heightened activity within the nursing home. When she was sat in a quiet room at mealtimes her screaming was even more intense.

Formulation

Failing eyesight had given rise to bewilderment and anxiety. A need for security.

Resolution

Gentle physical reassurances (stroking) by staff, but more especially from six residents whose occupational histories related to caring or looking after others.

Outcome

Significant diminution in noise making.

The final case of Betty (aged 69 years: diagnosis, probable vascular dementia) was complex and did not lend itself to rigorous behavioural analysis. Functional analysis established, however, the significance of her 'unobservable' personal variables and the purpose of her behaviour. Her individualised care plan was successful in meeting her need for security and occupation, thereby reducing the frequency and severity of her challenging behaviour.

The positive changes reported are testimony to the process of 'rementia' (Kitwood, 1989) contingent upon the recognition of 'the human value, worth and potential of people with dementia' (Woods, 1995). The adoption of a functional perspective enabled Moniz-Cook *et al,* (1999) to move away from the narrow confines of antecedents and consequences, and develop interventions based on hypotheses that addressed both the role of 'unobservables' and the influences of a broader time scale. These motivational dynamics cannot be overlooked as they are significant in helping us to plan appropriate psychosocial interventions.

Phenomena which potentiate or suppress behaviour–environment (situational) relationships are known as setting events (Emerson, 1993) and as such refer to the psychology of the person, their life history, their health status and the role of behavioural ecology (context), factors that may in themselves be complex phenomena temporally distant from the specific behaviour under scrutiny (as in the cases of, for example, Mrs O and Mr D). The potential advantages of incorporating the analysis of setting events into the analysis of challenging behaviour are considerable, for it indicates that, if interventions address the needs of the person and aspire to achieve the best person–environment fit we 'undercut the motivational basis underlying the challenging behaviour' (ibid). These are known as stimulus-based procedures, and are coming to replace the traditional behavioural predilection for 'management' of behaviour through the manipulation of consequences.

Functional displacement is an approach consistent with the notion that challenging behaviours may be conceptualised as meaningful acts and, consequently, intervention may consist of providing the person with functionally equivalent but more socially appropriate ways of meeting their needs. The encouragement of an alternative way of behaving may help us respond effectively to those comfortable remnants that are challenging to us. The objective is to establish a behaviour that serves the same motivational purpose but is no longer experienced as invasive. Clearly this can only happen if time is spent understanding the need that is fuelling the behaviour. Positive alternatives can then be suggested. Any similarities between interventions will only relate to the similarity of functions that the challenging behaviour serves. Hence it is not possible to make sweeping generalisations about interventions to be used (Samson & McDonnell, 1990).

The acquisition of functional equivalents can be seen as a variant of the constructional approach to intervention (Goldiamond, 1974). Rather than stop a behaviour, or reduce its frequency (for example, Birchmore & Clague, 1983), often without any regard to its motivation or meaning, the constructional approach may actually ignore the presenting problem and concentrate on building new behaviours. It again shifts a negative orientation to a positive one. The relationship between constructional interventions and functional displacement is transparent.

Moniz-Cook *et al*, (1999) used an approach based upon 'functionally equivalent' alternatives when working with Mary and Betty, as did Stokes (1996) with Mr D. In these cases efforts were directed towards finding ways of building on these individuals' strengths in order to help them find more constructive and acceptable alternatives to their challenging behaviours.

The effectiveness of psychosocial interventions based upon functional displacement is, however, dependent upon at least the following considerations:

1   The alternative response must be functionally equivalent to the challenging behaviour, not just socially appropriate (Emerson, 1993).

2   The alternative behaviour cannot be more 'effortful' (Carr, 1988).

3   Unless the functional equivalent alternative is a feature of the interaction between caregivers and the person with dementia, thereby allowing the new behaviour to be maintained or encouraged by the carer (as was the case with Mary), or we only make available the functionally equivalent response (in the case of Mr D, the flower beds were cleared of rocks, and a pile of large stones and rocks were made available for him to gather and store in a manner that was no longer destructive), the challenge is whether the new way of being can be learned. If it cannot, the existing behaviour will continue. As those with dementia have a significant learning deficit, this can have serious implications for the appropriateness of functional displacement as a means of working with challenging behaviour. As we have seen, recent work by Bird *et al*, (1995) has demonstrated that information can be retained if it is 'of practical value'. Similarly, Ikeda *et al*, (1998) have described the retention of emotionally significant experiences. While these reports of memory in dementia are of value, I believe that functional displacement may be of restricted utility when we are faced with challenging behaviour.

With the current developments in ecobehavioural and functional analysis, behavioural methods can no longer be seen as contrary to person-centred principles. As a result, our failure to help those who need our help may come 'not from inappropriate utilization of behavioural intervention but from the lack of application of such technology in situations that clearly warrant it' (La Vigna & Donnellan, 1986).

Sexual Needs
I believe our response (or, more accurately, lack of response) to the sexual needs of those with dementia warrants particular consideration.

As was discussed earlier (pp112–14), a dementing person remains a sexual being. Sexual feelings do not disappear just because memory and intellectual functions are fading. Kitwood & Bredin (1992) even consider the opposite may be true. Yet, in itself, this is not a challenge. Archibald (1995) maintains that it is 'a novel idea to see the expression of sexuality as a good thing, contributing to the individual's sense of identity and sense of personal well-being, as something which empowers the person'. The question is, how do we help them live with their sexuality? The answer is that, invariably, we do not, for while on the one hand we acknowledge their sexual needs, on the other we often fail to provide for its acceptable expression (Figure 6.1). As a consequence, we confront inappropriate and unwelcome sexual acts.

So how should we respond to the appearance of unacceptable sexual behaviour? With no prospect of a miraculous solution, I recommend the following step-by-step approach.

- Pinpoint precisely the behaviour so we are able to determine its nature. Is it sexual? If it is, is it inappropriate or does our revulsion reflect an ageist prejudice about sexuality in later life? Are we simply addressing sexual expression that is an affront to a carer's moral values?
- If we are confident a 'sexual problem' remains, how frequently does the behaviour occur? Archibald (ibid) advocates the methodology of behavioural analysis to establish frequency and to find out if there is a predictable pattern: that is, triggers (antecedents) and consequences. For example, sexual acting out has been associated with boredom. Our understanding will be further informed by the inclusion of a knowledge of the person ('the unobservables').
- If frequency is low, can the behaviour be tolerated? Having recognised that their sexuality is natural, can we be sensitive, understanding and discreetly preserve their dignity on the few occasions they act out?
- If frequency is high, but no pattern is revealed, could we be faced with sexual disinhibition as a result of neuropathology, for example frontal and temporal lobe lesions? If this is a possible explanation, ask for a neuropsychological examination.
- If a pattern is revealed that associates sexual acting out with intimate personal care, are the actions of caregivers provocative? Do carers mistakenly believe they are working with a person who is asexual? Assistance with self-care may provoke sexual arousal as the person who is being helped is unlikely to be aware of the true purpose of the intimate closeness and thus may easily misinterpret

the intention. So carers must always ask themselves whether their actions are compatible with the knowledge that the person remains an adult sexual being.

- If we cannot attribute the occurrence of sexual acting out to either neuropathology, an insensitive malignant social psychology, or the disinhibiting effects of drugs, such as alcohol and benzodiazepines, are we able to help the person express their sexual need in a manner that is acceptable to all concerned? Can we displace the inappropriate with an act that possesses functional equivalence?

- The person could be accompanied to their room and allowed to fondle their genitals or masturbate in private. The behaviour in this appropriate setting may be encouraged by the provision of provocative materials, such as magazines.

- If the person has a partner, can sexual relations be restored? An objective of person-centred understanding is to bring the individual back to life, to dispense with the notion that the person has departed ('He's not the person I married'), leaving behind a stranger who can be objectified and reduced to the status of symptoms. Armed with the knowledge that the person they have loved for years remains, can they find it in themselves to again be sexually intimate? This does not have to involve sexual intercourse, for sexuality is a complex amalgam of need implicating physical contact, emotional closeness and affection, as well as sexual satisfaction and relief. Is their partner able to respond to sexual feelings by kissing, holding hands or hugging, even though engagement in intercourse is denied?

    Partners may find this a very difficult and sensitive area to talk about. It lies within the private domain of life, and trust will need to be established before they feel able to communicate their feelings. They may abhor the prospect of surrendering to sexual demands. We must respect the needs of partners and appreciate that sexual relations may never be restored.

- It has been suggested that staff may address sexual needs through 'legitimate touch' (Archibald, 1995). This would include giving a hand massage or enabling a person to be held while dancing. While these are common-sense initiatives, the risk is that such engagement may be misunderstood, be experienced as provocative and result in heightened sexual arousal. If we embark upon such interventions, it is clear that we must be watchful of the consequences.

The ideas discussed here are limited in scope and do not provide easy options. Resolution may well be out of reach. As a result, we and they have to cope with a need that has not been met. When a woman lifts her skirt or a man starts to fondle his genitals we may distract them by introducing an activity of interest. Haddad & Benbow (1993b) suggest that clothing can be modified, for example if a man masturbates in public he can be provided with trousers without a zip. When carers observe or are subject to inappropriate behaviour they should not ignore, condemn or ridicule, but instead show tolerance and empathy and consider how gentle humour may defuse the situation. Respect is demonstrated by informing them that their behaviour is unacceptable, even though regard for them as a person remains. We must always be watchful that our communications are never demeaning, patronising or resonate 'infantilisation'.

Coping with a need that remains unmet is, in my experience the probable outcome. This is the reason for my assertion that we are in large part responsible for the appearance and maintenance of 'sexual problems'. We acknowledge their sexuality, but do little constructively to support a person who is suffering from a disability of intellect, not body, in their pursuit of sexual satisfaction. For example, we struggle with the ethical dilemma of condoning a person's attempts to start a sexual relationship with a fellow resident in care. Are the people involved competent to take part in sexual relations, that is, can they give informed consent? A valid concern, yet as Haddad & Benbow (1993a) assert, 'No diagnosis, not even dementia, is pathognomonic of incompetence to make decisions.'

These are controversial issues, but we cannot afford to turn away from them. If we do, the likelihood is that sedatives, anti-libidinal drugs and confinement, allied to expressions of disgust, will continue to be employed on the 'battlefield of sexuality and dementia' (Archibald, 1995) – actions designed to make *us* feel comfortable.

Person-Centred Working: Is it Evidence-Based?

Psychological interventions to resolve challenging behaviour are in their ground-breaking infancy, yet successes are reported time and time again.

The developing literature draws on anecdotal evidence, clinical casework and occasional single-case experimental studies (for example, Bird *et al*, 1995; Moniz-Cook *et al*, 1999). The limited number of empirical investigations has, however, led some to argue that our therapeutic work has yet to become evidence-based (Bleathman & Morton, 1994). If it was to be regarded as such this would encourage wider acceptance of psychosocial interventions (Moniz-Cook *et al*, 1999) as well as guarding against the rush to embrace fashionable but poorly validated approaches to working with people who are challenging.

The use of experimental procedures that demonstrate effectiveness within controlled research designs do, however, have a number of limitations. In general they are demanding of expertise and resources, both of which may be in short supply in care settings. But the most fundamental consideration is that the controlled experimentation of the 'scientific' method may in itself be inimical to the everyday practice of person-centred interventions.

Research and evaluation methodologies used in medical science and psychology have predominantly employed comparisons between groups of people to establish the validity of a therapeutic intervention. In a basic experimental design, 'subjects' would be randomly allocated to either a 'treatment' or 'control' group; the first group would receive the therapeutic intervention, and the second group would either not receive an intervention or would be given an alternative. Symptoms and/or performance would be measured before and after intervention, and a statistical comparison would be made of the results obtained. Any difference in the outcomes would then be attributed to the therapeutic intervention. It would be naïve to suggest that we could subject person-centred interventions to such controlled examination.

Resolution is enshrined within the quality of human relationships. It so often results from an empathic responsive way of being with others whose cognitive powers are failing, yet whose human needs remain unaltered. Rather than extolling the virtues of the scientific method and then decrying the absence of controlled research to demonstrate the suitability and effectiveness of our psychological interventions, what is probably required is an alteration in our appreciation of what is meant by 'therapy'. Through valuing the person, and communicating that value, we endeavour to understand the nature of their subjective experience and help them achieve well-being through the meeting of need. This results in changes to the interpersonal environment that are permanent arrangements, not time limited therapeutic interventions to be discontinued as soon as a goal is reached.

Our interventions are often micro-initiatives occurring on the most significant axis of the model of understanding (Figure 5.1), namely that between the person and those with whom they relate, in other words, ourselves. Hooper (1994) expresses it well: 'There was nothing clever about what we did, no special behavioural programmes ... Instead there was the formation of a therapeutic relationship between staff and patient essential for efficient care' – as Kitwood & Bredin (1992) said, 'person to person'. It is along this axis that we demonstrate empathy, acknowledge feelings and implement solutions. Perversely, traditional thinking on dementia promotes the health-built environment axis as being the most influential, when it has the least to offer in terms of resolution.

Our person-centred efforts do not warrant or lend themselves to controlled empirical experimentation. Let us consider the following attempts at resolution that are typical of the new culture of dementia care.

Michael

Challenging behaviour
Michael causes trouble by taking food off other people's plates.

Explanation
Michael is too restless to sit at mealtimes, even though hungry.

Need
Michael needs to eat in a socially acceptable manner.

Resolution
Carer makes Michael's meal into a sandwich, so he can eat as he walks about. (Kitwood & Bredin, 1992)

Jane

Challenging behaviour
Jane hoards household items and paper.

Explanation

Her world is changing for the worse. She is out of control. She feels lost, bewildered and unsafe. Hoarding is an effort to 'hold onto' what she has to maintain a sense of order when all around is chaos.

Need

Jane needs to feel secure.

Resolution

Provide Jane with a treasured possession to hold when she is anxious. Serve her favourite Earl Grey tea in the mug she has used for years. Play a piece of music that will resonate fond memories. Sit her by the window so she can enjoy the view she has known for years.

Susan

Challenging Behaviour

Susan attacks her husband when he gets into bed alongside her (see p68). David cannot cope. The family doctor advises, 'enough is enough'. The time has come for an admission to residential care.

Explanation

The destruction of most recent memories has, in Susan's eyes, rendered David a stranger. The image she has of her husband is of a man many years younger. Threatened and frightened, she tries to protect herself.

Need

Susan needs to feel safe and secure.

Resolution

David and Susan now sleep apart. She will not be getting up in the night to assault him spontaneously for her motivation was not dementia, but fear. No longer threatened, she sleeps soundly. Care at home continues for another 10 months.

The measure of success is the well-being of the person with whom we are interacting. This provides testimony to the effectiveness of our methods. Our subject matter is too immediate, too complex and impure to be measured by the standards of natural science, yet this need not be a cause for concern, for, while our data are less precise, conventional research that obtains 'noise-free knowledge in settings that are pure' (Kitwood, 1990) often falls prey to the principle of inconsequentiality. This principle states that 'the scientific acceptability of any technique of psychological investigation is inversely related to the importance of the question being asked'. Our questions pertain to the emotional health of real people whose vulnerability and suffering is often denied. We should expect our work to lack technical precision and methodological elegance. Certainly, at times there is scope for experimental designs using single case methodology (for example, Brooker *et al*, 1997; Moniz-Cook *et al*, 1999). This is a sound approach to demonstrate the effectiveness of interventions, yet such studies will always be few and far between. Their appearance in the literature will always be welcome, but true confidence in our therapeutic work must come from the daily experience of working with people whose frustrations and torment have been replaced by demonstrable improvements in well-being. It is these vignettes from real life that will inform the process of therapeutic practice and ensure that developments will have a direct bearing on the practicalities of care.

CHAPTER 11
Working with Unmet Need

A S WE SAW IN THE PREVIOUS CHAPTER, it is not always possible to resolve challenging behaviour. Needs cannot always be met. A model of understanding has been proposed that increases the prospect of solution, but it does not guarantee resolution. Alternatively, our challenge may be a person who is meeting their own needs, often living their 'comfortable ways', yet, as their actions are governed by the limits of their dementia, we experience disruption. Unfortunately, they are unable to acquire functionally equivalent behaviours that are appropriate and socially acceptable. In either instance the result of our inability to achieve resolution is that we must cope with the consequences.

The question that typifies the old culture of care is resurrected: 'How are we going to manage?' If challenging behaviour cannot be resolved, this is a legitimate question, for, if we cannot learn to tolerate and adjust, care will break down. This was the tragic outcome for Wendy. We could not resolve the complex web of underlying reasons for her toileting difficulty, and her husband was demonstrably unable to cope. She now lives in a nursing home with residents whose average age is over 30 years greater than her own.

In the absence of solution, psychological and practical strategies, some more effective than others, may enable us to manage better. Nowadays, however, our need to cope is grounded in two fundamental values. First, we are concerned with how we will manage only after full consideration has been given to ways in which the challenging conduct might be resolved and we have been found wanting. Second, we are working with a person whose needs must be respected and their actions understood, *not* symptoms of a disease to be managed and, if possible, eliminated. In other words, we do not lose sight of the person and revert to the language of problems. We acknowledge that for many our failure – for the challenge does not lie solely within them – will heighten their suffering and, even if we are able to cope with their conduct, this should not deflect us from our aspiration of resolution.

The Basic Principle

How we cope follows the same person-centred principles as resolution. In other words, whenever possible we refrain from giving prescriptive advice. The means to cope are shaped around the needs and strengths of all concerned. If we return to the case of Mr D, we responded to his need to be safe by making available a functionally equivalent response. There was, however, no successful resolution in terms of giving him what he had never possessed – peace of mind. Understanding him and his motivations enabled his wife to cope. Yet, despite her being better equipped emotionally to tolerate her husband's behaviour practical interventions were required:

- the gardens were tidied and restored to good order,
- a secure gate was placed at the end of the drive to prevent him gaining access to neighbours' gardens,
- the downstairs carpets were replaced, and
- whenever he went into the garden, his wife was advised to make sure that both the front and back doors were locked, thereby preventing him from wheeling his barrow into the house.

With the most damaging consequences of his conduct corrected, and with sensible measures in place, Mr D was able to continue his driven behaviour without interference. No longer was he confronted with demands to stop. With the consequences of his actions now contained, others could now be sensitive to his fears, 'reassuring him by touch and tone of voice that his actions were O.K.' (Stokes, 1996). Any sense of well-being was transient, but, as was discussed earlier, such supportive gestures are not diminished by their impermanent effect. The outcome of our intervention was to give Mrs D the confidence and commitment to care for her husband at home during the remaining months of his invasive behaviour.

Probably the most person-specific intervention I ever employed was with a man who would pace around his home throughout the day, trying to open doors. His wife was long suffering and just wished to have peace and quiet. We made no breakthrough with his behaviour beyond an acknowledgement that he felt confined. However, by talking to his wife we discovered that her husband had always enjoyed watching the main bulletin of the BBC News, to such an extent that their evening was structured around the programme. We video-recorded six of these half-hour bulletins including the distinctive signature tune. When either he was displaying a significant degree of agitation or his wife was particularly harassed, she would play the video and, on hearing the opening announcement and 'fanfare', he would sit down and watch the news. For him the outcome was a sense of familiarity and satisfaction, for his wife she gained respite without her husband having to attend day care.

The person and their context will always inform our efforts to structure a 'coping environment'. There are, however, general principles of good practice to consider too. First, we will examine interventions relevant to the specific challenges of wandering and aggression, and then critically examine the benefits of methods that are not specific to behaviour, namely distraction, behaviour modification, aromatherapy and medication.

Wandering

The provision of sensible security precautions helps reduce unnecessary risk and allows both family and professional carers to know that a crisis is less likely to occur. In the pursuit of peace of mind, I am not advocating a policy of protective custody, just sensible precautions to generate confidence among carers that it is safe for the person to walk.

Personal Information

Providing information such as name, address and telephone number on a card placed in a wallet, purse or pocket, or even on a label stitched inside their jacket or overcoat, may aid a speedy return home if a person is lost. It is important, however, that the information is carried in a way which does not 'signpost' the person as an individual at risk.

Alarms

These can be employed when professional caregivers have limited time to be watchful of the exits. Alarms can be triggered whenever a secured door is opened. Where such a system would be too intrusive, electronic tagging has been advocated. Triggered by a small tag fitted into the clothing of a person, the doors are open to all except those who are 'tagged'. However, there are certain issues and problems which need to be addressed when the use of electronic tagging is being considered (see Table 11.1).

The most significant reservation does not, however, relate to issues of implementation, but pertains to the ethical issue of 'tagging' someone. Because of the potentially fatal consequences, getting lost outside the home is one of the most worrying developments for carers. Tagging devices offer a solution, as do electronic transmitters that enable a person

Table 11.1 *Implications of electronic tagging*

Issue	Problem
The alarm must be unobtrusive so as not to distress either the person who is leaving or others in care.	Will there be sufficient staff to monitor a discreet alarm which may only be heard in the exit area or, if connected to a master console, in the office? If not, are mobile receivers available?
The electronic tag needs to be attached to clothing.	It is possible that the article of clothing could be removed by the person, and the alarm system thereby overcome. A danger is that 'tagging' can breed a false sense of security among staff.
A 'triggered' alarm system enables doors to be left 'open'.	A situation could arise wherein a 'tagged' person could lead out another resident with dementia who might remain outside unobserved and at risk.

to be tracked down if they are missing. While Marshall (1995) argues that technology 'is the shape of the future whether we like it or not', she accepts that we 'have to find a balance between the duty of care and freedom of choice'. The technology may benefit carers, but it is also associated with degrading and dehumanising treatment (Smith, 1994).

McShane *et al* (1994) propose that, in the right circumstances, tagging devices are desirable. If by leaving a building a person could be harmed (for example, knocked down by a car), as well as placing others at risk (for example, the driver involved in the accident), 'a degree of restriction of freedom is a price worth paying for the safety of the person and others'. McShane *et al* (ibid) propose a similar argument for tracking devices: 'if it is ethically proper to search for them, surely it would be proper to do so with the help of a tracking device'. It can even be argued that the use of this technology might enhance liberty by enabling a less restrictive form of care.

There is much to commend the view that a considered application of surveillance technology benefits the person with dementia, yet as Marshall (1995) declares, the need for safeguards to avoid abuse are equally compelling. These would include the following:

- operational definition of the 'problem',
- efforts made to resolve the behaviour,
- discussion with relatives and the appointment of an advocate,
- a decision to be made on the use of technology to 'manage' the behaviour,
- documentation to record performance and well-being of the person,
- specified time for review and who will be involved.

A simple alarm system that can be installed at the main entrance of a day centre or residential home connects the opening of the front door to the door-bell. Whenever the door is opened the bell sounds. Such a device is both unobtrusive and 'normal', and can be easily used within a person's own home. If the system is used at a day centre or in a continuing care setting where, for example, the main entrance is in constant use, the use of a digital code can prevent the bell ringing. The code is displayed by the door, and if it is punched in prior to the door being opened, the bell will not sound. As a person with dementia is unlikely to master the procedure (although those with fronto-temporal dementia may well be able to), when the bell sounds carers are alerted.

The introduction of a 'door-bell alarm' had an unexpected, albeit beneficial, outcome in the case of a man who persistently attempted to leave a day centre to go home – home being Belfast, a journey of over 300 miles! On his opening the front door, the bell rang. He would stop, look outside, see nobody there, scowl, and then, muttering to himself, step back inside and close the door!

Marshall (1995) also describes 'passive alarms' which can be placed under a mat beside the side of a bed or by interior doors to alert carers to the fact that a person is walking around the home. They are triggered when someone steps on them.

Locks

The locking of doors is not to be encouraged in continuing care establishments, but if the person with dementia lives at home the security of the front door does not constitute an infringement of personal liberty. If a carer is to be free of the need to mount a constant watch and have a sound night's sleep without worrying about whether a partner has slipped out of the house under the cover of darkness, locking the front door is an essential measure.

As people with dementia have difficulty in storing fresh information and learning new ways, a new lock on the door can be a significant barrier to leaving the house. The more complex the lock, the less likely it is that the problem will be solved. Locating a lock in an unfamiliar position, such as at the top or bottom of the front door, will make the opening of the door an even more complicated task. This is an alternative to a lock which is difficult to operate.

A safety measure used in care settings is to employ 'baffle handles' which need to be pulled simultaneously in opposite directions. These difficult-to-operate handles help to prevent the possible dangers of wandering, while providing maximum opportunity for physical activity within a designated area. Similarly, the use of digital locks which can puzzle the more able person with dementia who can overcome the 'baffle' system can be effective. Access to the establishment or unit can be 'open', but to leave the facility requires input of the digital code. Again, this can be displayed by the door for the benefit of visitors.

As with tagging and tracking technology, the introduction of locks and baffle systems raises concerns over individual liberty, but yet it can again be argued that such security initiatives can lead to a more relaxed, less repressive care regime. It is not the security of the exits that should warrant greatest debate, but what is happening behind the doors that are now secured. Such a policy encourages freedom of movement within the building rather than placing limitations on walking; it enables one-to-one activities as carers do not have to group people together in order to exercise a watchful eye; and it avoids the dedication of scarce staff time to surveillance duties by the main exit.

Secured doors can be integral to effective dementia care, but they should be employed judiciously, not be seen as an alternative to staff, and at all times the use of locks or similar barriers must be compatible with the requirements laid down by fire and safety regulations. The environment must ensure safety, but it cannot be the overriding theme of design.

Perimeter Boundaries

Securing the external perimeter can act as a fail safe response, or possibly an alternative to baffling or locking doors. If it is safe for someone to walk outside then restrictions on leaving a building have low priority.

While secure perimeters conjure up visions of high fences and imposing gates, this is far removed from what can be achieved with creative thought. At home, a bolt on the far side of the gate – best placed at the base – can be an insurmountable barrier. In continuing care establishments, as an alternative to fences, garden landscaping can deter people from leaving. People rarely walk across grass, let alone trample through flower beds, so a design that incorporates circular paths that meander through oases of colour and interest, raised flower beds, rose bushes with attractive trellis work behind and hedges can disguise the objective of establishing perimeter security.

Internal Design

Some people have noted the benefits of simple environmental changes. 'Wandering circuits' have been proposed (for example, Beck & Shue,

1994), whilst others have suggested that floor patterns, especially horizontal stripes before an exit door (Hewawasum, 1996), may reduce attempts to leave a home. Disguising a door by painting it the same colour as the adjacent walls will reduce its interest value and diminish the likelihood that it will be noticed.

At night a curtain or blind may be an effective means of disguise (see, for example, Dickinson *et al*, 1995). As this is not a constant environmental feature, the association between door and curtain is unlikely to be established. This is unlikely to work if the person lives at home, for it is over-learned knowledge that the front door is located at the end of a hallway.

Attaching a full-length mirror to internal doors will make recognition difficult (for example, Mayer & Darby, 1991). However, this design initiative needs to be balanced against the possibility of heightened disorientation, agitation and the risk of injury if the mirror is not properly secured.

All building and design adaptations to manage the risks and nuisance of wandering must avoid a sense of confinement. We are attempting to create a safe environment, not one that is unduly restrictive and thus a source of frustration. A distressing feature of dementia care is to see people banging on windows, persistently pulling at door handles or forlornly standing at a gate they cannot open. Their quality of life cannot be ignored just because they are no longer a cause for concern. 'It may be better to accept a small degree of risk than to hem a person in completely' (Kitwood & Bredin, 1992). This may sometimes conflict with the caution of relatives. Their worries cannot be dismissed. We need to talk about the unacceptability of physical and pharmacological restraint, and the need to provide a secure but caring environment with due regard for rights as well as the potential for risk.

Psychosocial Intervention
When somebody leaves a building, accompany them if at all possible. Nothing more is required. Just walk with them for a while. If they take your arm their wandering now becomes a stroll. If this approach is not feasible, and often this will be so, the following intervention involving two staff members can often work.

• Let the person walk away from the building for several moments (the length of time will be influenced by the range of safe distance).

- The first carer approaches the person and walks alongside them for a minute or so. No attempt is made to encourage them to return, unless the person wishes to do so. Striking up a conversation makes it a social happening.
- The second carer now approaches and asks both of them to return. If the person 'wandering' does not agree, the first carer says they will return shortly, at which point the second carer returns.
- A little while later, the first carer suggests they both go back. It is surprising how often the strategy works. The explanations for the method's effectiveness are likely to include the following:
  a trusting bond has been established ('holding');
  with the passage of time the motivation for leaving has been forgotten, the person may already be getting tired or cold;
  what faces them is unknown, what is behind is felt as known, and so it feels safer to return than to venture forth.

The use of these measures prevents confrontation and 'may be weighed against the alternatives, which are often psychoactive medication used for restraint' (Moniz-Cook, 1998).

Aggression

Carers often describe the difficulties they experience in coping with people who behave aggressively. This is understandable, for to be the victim of a physical attack or verbal abuse is distressing. Yet as has been revealed at length, aggressive acts rarely occur without reason (for example, Hooper, 1994). Thus prevention is always the favoured way of working. On occasions, however, acts of hostility are unexpected and inexplicable. Sometimes we let ourselves down and initiate an ambiguous, and possibly alarming, approach. In these instances we require knowledge and skill to respond appropriately, so preventing the episode escalating out of hand.

Bryan & Maxim (1994) provide useful guidance on how to work with a person who is shouting, swearing or accusing.

- try to stay calm,
- do not take the insults personally,

- back away, so that personal space is not infringed, and maintain eye contact (do not glare),
- give calm reassurance that all is well,
- while speaking slowly and gently, explain why you are with them,
- if verbal abuse persists, disengage and inform them that you will return later,
- attempt to determine the explanation for their abusive conduct, and then try again.

If carers are faced with a violent incident, the objective is to reduce the risk of injury to themselves, the person who is being aggressive and any bystanders, some of whom may be frail.

What Not to Do
1 Do not be confrontational.
2 Do not raise your voice.
3 Do not attempt to lead the person away or initiate any other form of physical contact, as such actions can easily be misunderstood.
4 Do not stay in their personal space (this varies from person to person, but at a time of distress a distance of about four feet is a useful estimate).
5 Do not attempt to approach from behind.
6 Do not corner the person as this will heighten feelings of threat and alarm.
7 Do not crowd them by calling for assistance.
8 Do not tease or ridicule.
9 Do not attempt to use restraints.
10 Do not show fear, alarm or anxiety, as this may serve to encourage the violent act and also cause agitation by demonstrating that it is not only they who are unable to cope, but you as well.

Recommended Practice
If we are to feel confident in our ability to cope with violent behaviour, we need to know what is expected of us at such times. The following responses, not all of which will be relevant in every episode, are essential for de-escalating violent situations.

1 Stay calm; this will demonstrate that you are in control.
2 Respect their personal space. This serves to reduce threat and enables carers to maintain a safe distance. Rather than facing the person directly, stand at an angle of 45 degrees. Ensure there are no items that can be reached which are likely to injure.
3 Try to convey reassurance by tone of voice, but also present as firm, so that boundaries of acceptable behaviour are appreciated. This is known as 'limit setting'.
4 If appropriate, and possible, ask or direct other people to draw back and not to interfere. Be concerned for those who are vulnerable.
5 Encourage them to talk rather than act out their anger. Engage eye contact and practise skills of active listening.
6 Ask the person what is troubling them. Try to identify why they are so angry. Voice tone should remain constant and not reflect irritation or tension.
7 Listen to what they say. Be accepting, not rejecting. Acknowledge their feelings, do not embark on correction and justification. Seek points of similarity rather than difference. Try to agree to something, thereby building the first small bond of co-operation. Focus on the 'here and now', rather than issues of the past.
8 Try to divert their attention if they remain angry. Give them the psychological room to move from their aroused state. Offer a way out. Provide alternatives to the behaviour. Keep options simple.

The objective of these actions is to defuse the situation. It is to be hoped that an empathic, responsive, but firm reaction will enable the person to calm down. At this point, someone else, if possible their keyworker, for they know them best, should talk to them. If they will accompany that person, this could happen somewhere quiet, away from the site of the incident. A gentle conversation in a tranquil area will be a 'holding' response to an upsetting experience.

The carer involved in the aggressive episode should be given the opportunity to talk through what happened with colleagues. There is no blaming, but a wish to learn from the episode. For example, how well did they respond to the person's anger and what are the underlying needs they must try to meet in order to prevent a similar episode in the future?

The Victim Who is at Serious Risk
If the person has lost control and risks injuring themselves, or if they are attacking somebody else who is vulnerable, caregivers need to respond effectively.

- No more than two carers are needed to intervene.
- Approach from the front, with speed but not haste.
- They should not be wearing anything visible which could be potentially harmful if it were to be grabbed.
- They need to speak in a calm, but matter-of-fact manner, requesting the person to stop or let go.
- A commentary should be provided to inform the person what is happening.
- If the assault continues, as a last resort and using minimal force, the carers should each take hold of an arm and disengage the person from the victim. No other physical contact is necessary. During this action the talking continues, reassuring the person and their victim that all will soon be well.
- Once the two are separated, the victim can be comforted by one of the carers.
- The other carer breaks away from the aggressor, respects their personal space and talks to them in accord with the guidelines for responding to a violent episode.

By following these recommendations on how to communicate with a person who is aggressive, and possibly violent, carers can avoid a traumatic confrontation at a time when everybody involved is feeling at their most vulnerable.

Non-Specific Interventions

Distraction
Distraction is often advised as a means of 'managing' a person's unwanted behaviour (as we have seen with aggression, or when a person is trying to leave a building). The challenge for us is that it is we who wish them to stop, not they. As a result, the activity we suggest must be at least as

attractive to them as their current behaviour, either because it is functionally equivalent or because it satisfies an equally significant need. If the objective is to be achieved, there is no doubt that we have to both understand the motivation for the behaviour and know them well to be able to suggest a rewarding and meaningful alternative.

Hooper (1994) described how her initial intervention with a 'violent' man was aided by the ease with which she could engage him in conversation about his children. The pen profile of 'Mr Smith' acknowledged that 'it was possible to distract him', yet this strategy will only ever be successful if the diversion relates to the biography of the person. Only then will we know what interests them, what they like to talk about and what they like to do. In other words, distraction must be person-centred.

Our request, for that is what it is, must be voiced as an enquiry; for example, 'Would you like …?, 'Shall we …?, 'How are your …? The request is simple, factual and relevant to who they are, sufficiently gentle to be non-threatening, but succinct enough to gain their attention and be understood.

The successful use of distraction can also only work if the care environment is 'resource-rich': not only must alternative activities be available, but there must be sufficient carers to devote time to being with people. Distraction cannot be over in the space of moments, for the likelihood is that the residual motivation will again energise the unwanted behaviour. Even when distraction is being employed as a technique to manage a critical incident, such as when someone is being aggressive, time is required to calm and soothe the person after the acute episode has passed.

Behaviour Modification
Nearly 20 years ago, Holden & Woods (1982) stated, 'In relation to dementia at least, behaviour modification is an extremely promising approach but as yet there remains a lack of convincing evidence for its effectiveness.' In the same year, Leng (1982) was less optimistic: 'the paucity of successful reports is not encouraging'. Twenty years on I believe it is true to say that behaviour modification is an intervention whose time never came. Bedevilled initially by therapeutic failure, today, the methodology is out of step with contemporary values.

Behaviour modification follows on from behavioural analysis and involves the application of operant conditioning principles and procedures to modify behaviour. Blackman (1981) defines behaviour modification as the changing of problem behaviour by using operant techniques to manipulate the environmental relationships which were controlling that behaviour. In essence, the immediate consequences of a behaviour are manipulated so that desired behaviours are rewarded (positive reinforcement) and unwanted behaviours are 'punished' through the withdrawal of reward. Success is therefore measured by the extent to which we can ameliorate the challenging behaviour. Stokes (1986a; 1986b; 1987a; 1987b) outlines the range of methods that can be either used or in the words of Perrin (1996), are 'rarely anything other than morally indefensible' (see Table 11.2). Unfortunately, therapeutic successes have been few and far between (for example, Birchmore & Clague, 1983). Patterson *et al* (1982) reported that people with cognitive impairment show slower and more limited progress.

An alternative behavioural methodology is to change those aspects of the environment that constitute the antecedents of a behaviour; this is known as 'stimulus control'. Fisher & Carstensen (1990) argue that this is the most appropriate approach to 'behaviour management'. Hussian (1981; 1982; 1988) and Hussian & Brown (1987) report the successful use of discriminative environmental cues (such as brightly coloured large cardboard shapes) paired with prompts and reinforcement to reduce noise making, inappropriate sexual conduct and wandering. For example, in the presence of a distinctive symbol a behaviour may be encouraged, but when faced with another design it will be discouraged. Bird *et al* (1995) successfully used cued recall (a large red stop sign) to reduce the number of times a woman walked into bedrooms to 'help' other nursing home residents.

Yet even these successes are tempered with caution. Fisher & Carstensen (1990) conclude that stimulus control is 'moderately effective for reducing the behaviour problems that accompany dementing disorders'. Bird *et al* (1995) acknowledged that, while adaptive behaviour change has been demonstrated, the 'rather equivocal outcomes raise questions about the utility of the work'. The failure to bear rich fruit of behaviour management techniques that manipulate environmental antecedents and/or consequences may implicate the profound learning deficit that characterises dementia and interferes with the acquisition of new information, despite efforts to make it relevant to 'case profiles'. If the

Table 11.2 *Techniques of behaviour modification*

Positive reinforcement	Akin to a reward, this is an event which, when presented to a person immediately following a behaviour causes that behaviour to increase in frequency.
Time out	The appearance of unwanted behaviour is followed by removal to a less reinforcing situation.
Response cost	Inappropriate behaviour is followed by the removal of a previously available positive reinforcer.
Restitutional over-correction	'Putting right' whatever aspect of the environment has been disturbed by an undesirable behaviour (restitution), in such a manner that it is restored to a better-than-normal state (over-correction).
Extinction	A previously reinforced behaviour is no longer reinforced, thereby causing the behaviour to reduce in frequency.

person cannot learn the relevance of a cue or remember the consequences of their actions then behaviour will not change. It may also reflect a lack of enthusiasm for the approach on the part of professional caregivers. It is often found that staff do not co-operate with the need for consistent application of prompts, reinforcement and placement of cues. The outcome is that learning gains dissipate. Long ago, Miller (1977) suggested that lasting improvements will require behaviour modification principles to be permanent features of the environment in order that necessary reinforcers for the maintenance of appropriate behaviour will always be present.

The essential core of the argument that these behavioural methods are of limited utility, and only warrant consideration when we are compelled to manage a person's behaviour, is not, however, founded solely on their failure to establish evidence of clear long-term success. It is because the methodology is inimical to person-centred values. Reference is made, not to the psychology of the person, but solely to the simplistic opinion that 'behaviour is lawfully related to the environment and so modifiable by changes within that environment' (Samson & McDonnell, 1990). There is little, if any, regard for the unobservable person variables that enable us to understand the person's world of meaning and need. For example, the nature of Max's difficulties enabled Bird *et al* (1995) to resolve his need to toilet, yet in their other case examples the objective was 'management of behaviour', not resolution. They acknowledged that 'Una' wished to help others, but the purpose of their behavioural intervention was simply to stop her from doing so. The objective was to diminish her problem behaviour 'to manageable levels'. There is no reference to resolving the challenging behaviour by constructing an alternative, socially appropriate functionally equivalent behaviour. It is as if Una's motivations were irrelevant, what was important was to control her behaviour. Yet an intervention has merit only if the person with dementia benefits at least as much as other people.

Similarly, Birchmore & Clague (1983), in their efforts to eliminate the undesirable behaviour of noise making demonstrate how the person is subordinate to the demands of behaviour management. Despite acknowledging that a woman who was both blind and dementing was shouting to compensate for sensory deprivation, as well as engaging in 'loud talking', the intervention was to provide her with the reinforcement of 'stroking' when she was quiet. In other words, when she 'felt' her under-stimulation and shouted, she was ignored, yet when she was quiet and thus not demonstrating the effects of her impoverished surroundings (we can surmise that at these times she may have been content while attending 'the theatre of her mind'), her back was pleasantly stroked. If she then communicated with that person ('loud talking'), 'we stopped stroking her ... when she began to talk'. In other words, her need for human contact was denied. This illustrates why behaviour modification is anathema to the practice of person-centred care. Although the presence of the person may be acknowledged, the methodology does not take the individual's needs as its driving force.

Present-day behavioural interventions (described in Chapter 10) are very different. These employ functional analysis to establish meaning and purpose, are constructional in approach and address the need for resolution, not management. It is not surprising that the increased understanding that this methodology gives is likely to lead to a more successful intervention than behavioural approaches which concentrate on changing aspects of the environment in which a person is living.

This is not to say that behaviour management is never to be considered. A basic, yet sensible suggestion is to 'avoid unwittingly reinforcing unwanted behaviour by paying it unnecessary attention' (Haddad & Benbow, 1993b). Time and time again this is what is observed, not because understanding is being sought or constructive approaches are being adopted, but simply to 'fuss' and rebuke. This adds to the distress of the moment, but for those few in our care who retain the ability to recall and reason, undue attention may serve to encourage the dysfunctional behaviour. We do not ignore, for that could result in escalation and a corresponding deterioration in the person's behaviour. Also such inaction does nothing to help us resolve the challenge before us. Instead, our attention must be considered and with clear purpose.

A behaviour management approach may also be a psychosocial option if, by doing nothing, the person is, for example, placing themselves or others at risk. Bird *et al* (1995) report that 'Una' was sometimes attacked when she interfered with the personal belongings of others. While establishing a more constructive and acceptable alternative behaviour would have been desirable, for Una was now denied an opportunity to meet what was to her some kind of significant need, if this was not possible then teaching her the association between the cue and 'safe' behaviour was a valued intervention. It is a technique which, if intelligently tailored to the person's circumstances, may avoid the introduction of pharmacological control. And this is where the methodology is best placed in the new culture of dementia care – a psychosocial act of last resort with modest prospects of success.

Aromatherapy

From the old to the new. Whereas behaviour management resonates with images from the old culture of care, the addition of aromatherapy to psychosocial interventions is a modern development.

Aromatherapy has many champions in dementia care. Aroma diffusers are used in Snoezelen rooms as part of the multisensory experience known as 'sniff and doze therapy' (Benson, 1994). It is suggested that exposure to a multisensory environment helps stimulate those who are withdrawn and calms those who are agitated. In a study by Dowling *et al* (1997), Snoezelen sessions were found to reduce socially disturbed behaviour, such as being objectionable to others, hoarding useless items, shouting and swearing.

Examining the effect of aromatherapy in isolation, West & Brockman (1994) report how the technique improved one man's nocturnal disturbance and 'compulsive daytime activity', while Burleigh & Armstrong (1997) assessed whether the use of aromatherapy oils could reduce challenging behaviours in people with severe dementia. Essential oils were used in baths, applied to pillows and massaged on the hands, neck, face and shoulders. Over a 12-week period, challenging behaviours were significantly reduced in five of the seven people in their study. However, the two men revealed an increase in challenging behaviour following the introduction of aromatherapy massage. This may have been the result of their reacting adversely to intimate touch and indicates that the practice of aromatherapy must consider not only contraindications and potential for allergic reactions, but also the issue of cultural acceptance. It also needs to be recognised that effects may well vary considerably between individuals. Using a robust single-case research design, Brooker *et al* (1997) demonstrated that it was just as likely for disturbed behaviour to increase following exposure to aromatherapy and massage as it was for the technique to result in demonstrable benefits. Such idiosyncratic responses make clear that complementary therapies are not a general panacea. It is even possible that essential oils may have a different effect on specific challenging behaviours.

These are early days, but it already appears that the considered use of aromatherapy has benefits for some, although not all, people who are challenging. The optimism of a few years ago is being replaced by balanced opinion and questions that remain unanswered. We need further research to inform and illuminate our practice. Only then will we have a sound knowledge base to help us identify who is likely to derive the greatest benefit. As Moniz-Cook (1998) comments, progress cannot be built on wishful thinking and 'anecdotal reports'.

Medication
This is the true last resort, yet so often not only a common response to challenging behaviour in dementia (Tobiansky, 1995), but the first method of intervention (MacDonald & Teven, 1997). Struble & Sivertsen (1987) observed that nurses might use psychotropic drugs within five to 15 minutes for residents who were seen as aggressive or antisocial. Year after year reports are published documenting the widespread symptomatic use of major tranquillisers (neuroleptics) to control agitation, aggression and other 'problem behaviours', use that can often be seen as evidence of misuse (Taft & Barkin, 1990). Drugs have become little more than chemical constraints, prescribed to make a person more manageable. 'The trouble is, it makes them less of a person' (Kitwood & Bredin, 1992).

It is not even as if there is methodologically sound evidence for the use of neuroleptics and other psychotropic medications in the management of troublesome behaviours in dementia (Schneider & Sabin, 1994). Ballard (2000) reports that while there is symptom improvement in 60 per cent of cases following the introduction of neuroleptics, 40 per cent improve after placebo treatment! Patel & Hope (1993) note that when major tranquillisers are used to manage aggressive behaviour, 'they may lead to worsening of the behaviour'. Yudofsky *et al* (1990) go so far as to recommend that neuroleptics be used in the management of chronic aggression only if there is evidence that psychosis is a factor causing the behavioural disturbance. Sunderland & Silver (1988) report, however, that neuroleptics have a role in the management of dementia when used at *low* dose. There is no evidence that polypharmacy is effective (Ballard, 2000). Tobiansky (1995) warns that older people with dementia may be more sensitive to the common side-effects of neuroleptics, which include sedation, postural hypotension, constipation and movement disorders known as 'extrapyramidal side effects'. Dementia with Lewy bodies (DLB) is characterised by exaggerated adverse responses to standard doses of neuroleptic medication (a neuroleptic sensitivity syndrome). It is not surprising that Wattis (1990) concludes that 'Sedative medication is only one of a range of alternative approaches and, because of the possibility of unwanted effects, should be reserved till other measures have been tried and found to be ineffective.'

If psychotropic medication is prescribed for symptomatic use, Wattis (ibid) advises the principle of minimal medication: 'It is essential that the minimum number of drugs are prescribed in the lowest effective dose for the shortest time necessary to produce the desired effects.' Tobiansky (1995) identifies the need for medication reviews following the commencement of treatment, while Kitwood & Bredin (1992) emphasise that carers can make a valuable contribution at such times. It is not for the psychiatrist or general practitioner to assume they are the fount of all knowledge. It is so often the case that those furthest from the person and their challenging behaviour believe they know the most, when they in fact know the least. It is those who are closest who know what is happening on a day-to-day basis, not those who are around for a very short time. Document the positive and negative effects of the medication, describe accurately, not loosely, and have confidence that, while you may not be an expert on medication, you are the expert on the person in your care (Kitwood & Bredin, 1992) and somebody must be the advocate for those who cannot speak for themselves.

CHAPTER 12

The Challenge of Confusion

W E END OUR PSYCHOLOGICAL EXAMINATION of challenging behaviour by again entering the world of confusion. In some ways this presents us with our greatest challenge. I have not always thought this, for can we not collude and practice reality orientation to minimise the distressing effects of confused behaviour? The real challenge is to address those who are suffering in the 'here and now' as they try to meet, or face up to the frustration of their needs. Over a decade on from our appreciation that needs motivate much that challenges us in dementia, our therapeutic successes encourage me to believe that resolution is a realistic aspiration for many people who are labelled as 'disruptive', 'difficult' or 'a problem'. Needs can be identified, motivations understood, potential established and resolution attempted. However, what about those whose needs are experienced within the psychological reality of years past? How do we bring peace of mind to a person who knows her children are lost, her mother is waiting and they are going to be late for work? How do we meet their needs? We cannot, all we can do is alleviate their torment. In essence we are again working with unmet need. Hence much that was conveyed in the previous chapter is relevant to the way we relate to the person who is confused. We need, however, to consider the merits of approaches that are specifically relevant to confusion: reality orientation, time-shift collusion and validation.

Reality Orientation

'There can be few people working in dementia care who have not come across Reality Orientation (RO)' (Woods, 1994). Its origins can be traced back to the work of Dr James Folsom at a Veteran's Administration hospital in the late 1950s (Taulbee & Folsom, 1966; Folsom, 1967, 1968). By the mid 1960s practice developments had led to the distinction between 'informal' or '24-hour' RO, on the one hand, and structured, time-limited RO groups, on the other.

Growth in the use of RO throughout the 1960s and 1970s (not only with people with dementia, but also with those suffering from mental illness and the effects of institutionalisation) led Hussian (1981) to consider RO to be the major psychological intervention employed in dementia care in the United States. A similar expansion in the use of RO occurred in the United Kingdom between 1975 and the early 1980s. Bird *et al* (1995) refer to 'the heyday of reality orientation'. However, 'interest began to wane as it all too quickly became clear that here was no miracle cure' (Woods, 1994). Miller (1987) reported on the limitations of RO, while Dietch *et al* (1989) wrote of the 'adverse effects'. This led to Woods (1994) raising the question, 'Does RO have a place in dementia care in the 1990s?' And beyond?

Nowadays, 'formal' RO groups are best seen as social gatherings whose benefits, whether these be interpersonal or cognitive, are rapidly lost once the session ends. This is only disappointing if we are expecting lasting improvement. The human contact and social exchange experienced within the groups are to be valued in their own right. These sessions may be the only time during the day that people with dementia are in meaningful contact with carers. The benefits of 'feeling wanted, esteemed and able to contribute can have remarkable effects' (Holden, 1990c). This raises the question, if it is social needs that are being met, why structure them as RO groups? Why talk about the date, the weather and the diary of the day? Why not talk about anything and everything? This does happen. Holden (ibid) sees formal RO as including 'a wide range of activities, such as reminiscence, exercise and games'. Yet the emphasis on orientation information remains. However, this is not so much for the benefit of those with dementia, but is instead of greater value to staff leading the groups. It is not easy to communicate at length with people who have dementia. As the well of enthusiasm runs dry, conversation becomes sparse. The RO format provides structure and purpose and thus helps to maintain staff motivation.

'In the 1990s RO will be a 24-hour approach … reducing confusion, minimising excess disabilities and promoting independent action' (ibid). This is contemporary RO in practice, helping people to appreciate their whereabouts and the events around them. Caregivers present accurate and detailed information in everyday conversation and provide a commentary on what is happening as they engage with the person. 'Confused, rambling speech is corrected or ignored.' From this account of RO it is clear there are two elements to the practice. It is designed to improve orientation and also alleviate confusion (Dietch *et al*, 1989), yet the same approach of informing and correcting is being applied to two different subjective phenomena. Herein lies the problem.

Orienting people to their environment, both social and built, is a valued exercise. Common sense dictates the need to use environmental cues (for example, pathfinder arrows, colours and symbols) as well as verbal orientation to help them find their way. The challenge is that they do not remember. They do not retain what they are told, nor can they remember the purpose of the environmental designs. A cue to assist recall is useless unless the person learns the association between the cue and the information it is supposed to convey. Without learning this, the cue has no meaning: a red door is just a red door (Bird *et al*, 1995). Though some people eventually learn the cue-information association, most do not. Improvements in verbal orientation have been demonstrated (for example, Hanley *et al*, 1981; Woods, 1983), but the results of RO in counteracting the more disabling consequences of disorientation have been generally disappointing (Bleathman & Morton, 1994). Hanley *et al* (1981) and Gilleard *et al* (1981) showed that environmental cues and intensive orientation training did improve behavioural functioning, as did a single case study reported by Lam & Woods (1986), but the weight of evidence is that general behaviour does not improve. Overall, lasting benefits are minimal and largely restricted to verbal orientation.

This relative failure to address the challenge of disorientation has led professional caregivers to become cynical and apply the techniques of RO in a rote, uninspired manner (Morton & Bleathman, 1988; Dietch *et al*,

1989). They complain that it is tedious reminding people of the day, where they are, where to go and what is happening next; and what is the point, anyhow: 'RO doesn't work.'

It is clearly evident that some of the information communicated has little relevance to the daily life of a person with dementia. If every day is unchanging then it is apposite to ask why they need to know the day of the week. RO cannot be divorced from life quality. The fundamental criticism of RO is, however, that it fails, yet what would be the measure that affirmed, 'RO does work'? What caregivers are saying is that those with dementia do not remember, yet how can they? As a result of pervasive and profound memory impairment, disorientation is a defining characteristic of dementia. Unless a person is at the beginnings of the disease process, it does not matter how often they are told, they will never remember. A misconception clearly reigns.

RO is a prosthetic therapy. It cannot resolve the underlying inability to learn. Prosthetic interventions compensate for what has been lost or damaged. We have no problem with physical prostheses, if a person needs a hearing aid, dentures or a walking aid, these are provided. After a period of use, we do not take them away, expecting the person to have been restored to their previous self. If we see a man affected by physical frailty progressing towards the toilet holding onto a handrail, and then, having toileted successfully, returning to his chair in the lounge, again clutching the handrail, we would not say that he is now able to toilet independently, and remove the handrail. We are human handrails continuously presenting the person with information relating to their physical and social surroundings (Holden, 1987). We support their finding their way around the home with prompts and reminders; we regularly inform them of our and others' identities and we let them know what is happening around them. They may not learn, but they are still able to achieve the valued goal of 'assisted independence' through the creation of this prosthetic environment. Bignall (1996) describes how the introduction of orientation designs improved way finding, reduced incidents of inappropriate urinating and helped foster independence. However, 'the most important aspect of the success of the project was the enthusiastic and positive attitudes of all the staff'.

I do not view the principle objective of RO as comprising the promotion of independent action, for I do not regard RO as being solely a prosthetic memory therapy. RO is seen by some 'as a dehumanizing behaviour modification technique, solely preoccupied with targeting symptom management' (Bleathman & Morton, 1994) and is thus seen as fitting ill in the new culture of dementia care. In response to this criticism, I believe RO can be reinterpreted so that it is sensitive to the subjective experience.

Those with dementia are lost and bewildered, we are not. We know they are safe and well, they feel only the unknown. It is the purpose of RO to provide reassurance to those who are suffering the distress of disorientation. We are there to salve troubled emotions and calm their anxieties by replacing 'not knowing' with awareness. Even if we do not observe demonstrable improvement in daily living performance, the knowledge that we have identified with their subjective pain and for valued moments promoted well-being means that RO is worth practising. The person who is frightened by the strangeness before them does not wish to hear how enjoyable the day will be. Their fear needs to be acknowledged, the accuracy of their observations affirmed. This is the domain of person-centred RO, addressing the subjective experience of dementia, informing and thereby emotionally supporting them at times of distress. Certainly, they will be back again, as troubled as before. But this is the nature of dementia. Their behaviour can be demanding and, at times, irritating. Yet I believe that, if carers appreciate they are attempting to meet emotional needs, rather than just seeking to improve behavioural functioning, they may be more inclined to embrace RO as an empathic approach that respects the whole person and hence remains 'part of the range of options available in dementia care' (Woods, 1994).

However, we have yet to consider the relevance of RO to confusion. Here the frustration of caregivers is not that those with dementia do not learn, but that they do not believe. When carers are faced with a person's desperate pleading for partners, parents or children, or their demands to go home, the first principle is to determine whether the person is confused, or perhaps using their language as a metaphor for needs that can be met in the 'here and now'. If we are confident that they are truly communicating a time past, the challenge is that they will not accept our reality. We engage in reality confrontation. 'It seems so confrontational and possibly distressing to attempt to orientate them to our current reality' (ibid). This turn of events is not surprising for we now appreciate that their reality is a world of conviction, not belief. If our reality is not amenable to correction, how can theirs be?

As we saw in Chapter 4, their subjective reality is known and maintained by psychological dynamics that thwart our efforts to inform and correct: efforts that are further undermined by our lack of credibility. Despite our caring roles and professional titles, to the person with dementia we are not known. Our intentions are puzzling, our actions disturbing. Even their own families are rendered unknown. Trust is lost. To be assured by a stranger that this is your home, your children are safe or your partner is dead, when you know it is not so is unlikely to result in 'participation in present reality' (Feil, 1992).

Yet is confrontation inevitable? The answer is 'no'. It is often observed that, as carers become exasperated, they apply RO in an insensitive and, on occasions, brutal manner. They practise on a cognitive level, focusing on facts and logic. Dietch *et al* (1989) illustrate how bringing a person into the 'here and now' can result in emotional upset:

- an 84-year-old woman who said her son was seven years old reacted with fury when told he would have to be much older;
- an 85-year-old woman, when told her parents are dead, 'becomes upset, cries and experiences urinary frequency with incontinence';
- a 74-year-old man, when told his brother is dead, becomes agitated, angry and then withdraws into himself.

On these occasions the approach is misapplied. There has been a disregard for feelings and a loss of regard for the person. There is preoccupation with cognitive deficits and an objectification of the individual. We must learn that the principle of showing respect for the individual and demonstrating empathy for their feeling experience take 'primacy over any approach or technique' (Woods, 1994). Caregivers need to appreciate the need for well-being and then decide when, how or even *if* they should be oriented to present reality. Yet what if our judgement is that RO, even when communicated with humanity, will not only fail to improve awareness, but is likely to cause distress. What are we to do? Woods (1992) states that 'the golden rule in RO is never to agree with what the person says if it is clearly wrong', an understandable assertion if we are working with someone's disorientation, but who is to say who is right or wrong when two realities coincide – ours and theirs?

Time-Shift

Holden (1990c) advocates a hybrid of RO and distraction known as 'time-shift' when communicating with a person who steadfastly holds onto their reality. If they demand to go home to be with their mother, it may be appropriate to say, 'It must have been nice when your mother was at home with you. What was she like?' The past tense is used with care, acknowledging their feelings and yet correcting the time perspective. In due course, the objective of the communication is to bring the person into present reality by saying 'You must miss her very much.'

Holden (ibid) acknowledges that the approach 'might be resented'. The technique is, however, a welcome addition to our therapeutic armoury, but the prospect of avoiding confrontation must be tempered with realism, if not caution. Furthermore, if the final step of reality awareness is likely to produce trauma, I have found that simply reminiscing, and hence achieving an accurate time-shift, may be both rewarding and may reduce the motivation to 'search'. We conclude the conversation with reference to the 'joys of nostalgia' and either move on to an unrelated topic or disengage.

Collusion

When we agree with a person's perception of reality, that is collusion. Dietch *et al* (1989), in their description of Validation Therapy (Feil, 1967; 1992) provide examples of collusion:

- 'At times she asks the staff when her son is going to visit next. Some staff members tell her that her son will be visiting later in the day.'
- '... the patient has refused to eat while she insists on knowing whether her mother fixed the meal. Staff have found that she will only eat if told that her mother did indeed prepare the food.'

Collusion has a role to play in dementia care, but in a way similar to that proposed for behaviour management. It is a psychological response of last resort when working with confusion. The approach may reassure or soothe a person who is distressed when we know, for example, that RO would precipitate an extreme reaction, or distraction would be ineffective. Unfortunately, we often see collusion employed as a general way of relating to a person who is confused. It is a means by which carers can extricate themselves from challenging interactions by simply agreeing with demands or requests, knowing full well their words will be forgotten within moments:

'I must go home. Take me home'.
'I can't at the moment, I'm busy. But I'll be back in a minute, and you can go then.'

The carer can move on and the confused person is placated, but look how little time has been devoted to meaningful communication. The relationship is founded on deceit and deception. If we truly hold the belief that a person with dementia is as we are, then this is a malignant interpersonal response. When all else fails, there may be occasions when we resort to collusion, but malign agreement should not be a characteristic of dementia care, the motivation for which is our need for a 'quieter life', while their social experience is affected by 'treachery' (Kitwood, 1990).

Validation
While it would be wrong to dismiss RO as the mechanistic communication of information and instruction, 'it is not a therapy aimed at uncovering, understanding and reflecting ... feelings' (Stokes & Goudie, 1990). Exponents of RO have addressed the criticism that the approach is devised to reorient the person to their current reality (Folsom, 1967) by going beyond traditional boundaries (for example, Holden, 1990c) to give the impression that 'RO is a generic term covering almost any kind of psychological intervention' (Miller, 1987). This gives rise to the real danger that RO loses its precision and we lose sight of a great deal that can be gleaned from the experience of applying RO.

Although RO has been reframed so it can take its place within the tradition of humanistic psychology, the emphasis of RO remains the communication of accurate information and the correction of confused speech. Validation Therapy (VT) is very different. VT was developed by Naomi Feil at the Montefiore Home for the Aged in Cleveland, Ohio (Feil, 1967). Deemed as appropriate for those with 'late onset dementia' (Feil, 1992), VT disputes the need to orientate and argues that we accept 'whatever reality they are in, in order to ease distress and restore self-worth' (Morton & Bleathman, 1991). It does not concern itself with factual errors, but acknowledges that the feelings are true and these are the material for therapeutic intervention. 'Validation works so much on a feeling level' (de Klerk Rubin, 1994). A woman knows her children to be young and missing, we know them as adults who are safe and well. She is objectively wrong, but subjectively there is no right or wrong. This is her unquestioning experience and her feelings are real. The acceptance of the reality and 'personal truth' of another's experience is known as validation (Kitwood, 1996). It is at this point that we need to distinguish validation from VT.

The theory of VT (see Morton, 1999 for a critique) is incoherent and unconvincing (Morton & Bleathman, 1995), offering little to our understanding of dementia (Goudie & Stokes, 1989; Stokes & Goudie, 1990). Despite, rather than because of, VT's theoretical aspirations, Feil's methods of working have enabled us to appreciate the benefits of validation when practised with confused older people. While validation is by no means unique to VT, being common to all humanistic therapies, including resolution therapy, Feil employed validation to show that confusion was no barrier to meaningful communication. The focus of interaction was the other person's subjective experiences.

As she rejected the cognitive and behavioural goals of RO, Feil combined a respect for the subjectivity of the confused person with an increased concern for their emotional well-being. Through empathic listening we discover their reality in order to make emotional contact (Wetzler & Feil, 1978). Factual inaccuracies are disregarded and the emotional implications or accompaniment of what is being said assume great significance: 'In verbalising the fantasy or inner reality, individuals gained a feeling of gratification, of being understood, and a sense of self in the knowledge that their world was meaningful and acceptable' (Feil, 1972). We need to be sensitive to their feelings of anger, frustration, sadness and despair. 'If we do not accept these feelings and allow others to express them, we are giving them the message that we do not take these feelings seriously, that the feelings are not real' (Kitwood & Bredin, 1992).

If a person with dementia is wanting to go home to their mother, we do not correct or collude, but instead we try to get a sense of the emotion that is coming across with the words and empathise with their feelings of, say, worry and anxiety. As Morton & Bleathman (1995) exclaim, we are 'liberated to build human relationships with those who are in the process of becoming starved of the opportunity for such contact'.

Unlike resolution therapy, where meaningful and empathic interpersonal contact is the vehicle to appreciate the changes required to meet someone's needs, validation is the necessary change when working with confusion. Acknowledging the reality of their feelings and providing empathic responses that validate these emotions enables the person to feel the warmth of acceptance. In the beginning they are angry and agitated. We present with calm reassurance. I find it is often best not to mention their confused demands and pleadings but, instead, focus on the feeling tone. It is this that we reflect and explore, and as we do so their failing memory becomes our ally. The initial motivation for their distress slowly fades, to be replaced by the quality of the therapeutic interaction. Where there was once isolation and panic, that person now finds themselves relating to somebody:

- who smiles,
- whose manner is gentle and respectful,
- whose tolerance affirms their worth, and
- who looks with unfrightened eyes at elements of which they are fearful (Rogers, 1980).

Ill-being is replaced by relative well-being and the episode becomes a 'holding' experience. This rarely happens with RO. Even though modern RO values the person and recognises their capacity for well-being, during discourse even gentle attempts to correct act as prompts, reminding the person of the source of their fears and frustrations. As a result, well-being is compromised as their 'confused' motivations remain accessible to awareness. Validation is more likely to achieve therapeutic gains because their 'error' is allowed to wither on the vine as our non-corrective responses concentrate instead on the expression and sharing of emotions, emotions that will be positively affected by the experience of validation.

Validation does not ensure success. It most definitely does not constitute a remedy to be used at all times with all people. Nor is it meant to replace or compete with other methods of working with confusion. What it is is an empathic psychosocial intervention that helps us get closer to the experience of those whose reality is very different from our own and for whom there is no true resolution. As ever, we endeavour to understand, we affirm the value of effective communication and continually search for means to nurture emotional well-being: actions that are person-centred, not prescribed, for, with the subjective experience of dementia guiding our practice, how can it be otherwise?

References

Albert SM, 1992, 'The Nature of Wandering in Dementia: a Guttman Scaling Analysis of an Empirical Classification Scheme', *International Journal of Geriatric Psychiatry* 7, pp783–7.

Alexander C et al, 1977, *A Pattern Language,* Oxford University Press, New York.

Alzheimer A, 1907, 'Über eine Eigenartige Erkrankung der Hirnrinde', *Allgemeine Zeitschrift fhr Psychiatrie,* 64, pp146–8.

Alzheimer's Disease Society, 1995, 'Services for Younger People with Dementia', *A Report by the Alzheimer's Disease Society,* London.

American Psychiatric Association, 1980, *Diagnostic and Statistical Manual of Mental Disorders,* 3rd edn *(DSM-III),* American Psychiatric Association, Washington, DC.

Anthony-Bergstone CR, Zarit SH & Gatz M, 1988, 'Symptoms of Psychological Distress Among Caregivers of Dementia Patients', *Psychology and Ageing* 3, pp245–8.

Archibald C, 1995, 'Sexuality and Sexual Needs of the Person with Dementia', Kitwood T & Benson S (eds), *The New Culture of Dementia Care,* Hawker Publications, London.

Arie T, 1987, 'Personal Communication', *Norman A, Severe Dementia: The Provision of Longstay Care,* Centre for Policy on Ageing, London.

Bailey D, Kavanagh A & Sumby D, 1998, 'Valuing the Person: Getting To Know Their Life', *Journal of Dementia Care* 6, pp26–27.

Baldwin RC, 1997, 'Depressive Illness', Jacoby R & Oppenheimer C (eds), *Psychiatry in the Elderly,* 2nd edn, Oxford University Press, Oxford.

Ballard C, 2000, *Managing Behaviour and Psychological Symptoms in Dementia,* Oxford University Press, Oxford.

Barlow DH & Hersen M, 1984, *Single Case Experimental Designs: Strategies For Studying Behaviour Change,* Pergamon, Oxford.

Barnes R & Raskind M, 1980, 'Strategies of Diagnosing and Treating Agitation in the Aged', *Geriatrics,* 3, pp111–19.

Barnett E, 1995, 'Broadening Our Approach to Spirituality', Kitwood T & Benson S (eds), *The New Culture of Dementia Care,* Hawker Publications, London.

Barrowclough C & Fleming I, 1986, *Goal Planning With Elderly People,* Manchester University Press, Manchester.

Beck CK & Shue VM, 1994, 'Interventions for Treating Disruptive Behaviour in Demented Elderly People', *Nursing Clinics of North America* 29, pp143–55.

Bell J & McGregor I, 1995, 'A Challenge to Stage Theories of Dementia', Kitwood T & Benson S (eds), *The New Culture of Dementia Care,* Hawker Publications, London.

Benson S, 1994, 'Sniff and Doze Therapy', *Journal of Dementia Care* 2, pp12–14.

Bergmann K & Jacoby R, 1983, 'The Limitation and Possibilities of Community Care for the Elderly Demented', *Elderly People in the Community: Their Service Needs,* HMSO, London.

Berlyne DE, 1960, *Conflict, Arousal And Curiosity,* McGraw-Hill, New York.

Berlyne DE, 1966, 'Curiosity and Exploration', *Science* 153, pp25–33.

Berrios G & Brook P, 1985, 'Delusions and the Psychopathology of the Elderly with Dementia', *Acta Psychiatrica Scandinavica* 68, pp263–70.

Bignall A, 1996, 'Look and Learn: Designs on the Care Environment', *Journal of Dementia Care* 4, pp12–13.

Birchmore T & Clague S, 1983, 'A Behavioural Approach to Reduce Shouting', *Nursing Times,* 20 April, pp37–9.

Bird M, Alexopoulos P & Adamowicz J, 1995, 'Success and Failure in Five Case Studies: Use of Cued Recall to Ameliorate Behaviour Problems in Senile Dementia', *International Journal of Geriatric Psychiatry* 10, pp305–11.

Birkel RC, 1987, 'Toward a Social Ecology of the Home-Care Household', *Psychology and Ageing* 2, pp294–301.

Birkett DP, Desouky A, Han L & Kaufman M, 1992, 'Lewy Bodies in Psychiatric Patients', *International Journal of Geriatric Psychiatry* 7, pp235–40.

Blackman D, 1981, 'The Experimental Analysis of Behaviour and Its Relevance to Applied Psychology', Davey G (ed), *Applications of Conditioning Theory,* Methuen, London.

Bleathman C & Morton I, 1994, 'Psychological Treatments', Burns A & Levy R (eds), *Dementia,* Chapman & Hall Medical, London.

Bowen DM, Allen SJ, Benton JS, Goodhardt MJ, Haan EA, Palmer AM, Sims NR, Smith CCT, Spillane JA, Esiri MM, Neary D, Snowdon JS, Wilcock GK & Dowison AN, 1983, 'Biochemical Assessment of Serotonergic and Cholinergic Dysfunction and Cerebral Atrophy in Alzheimer's Disease', *Journal of Neuropsychiatry* 41, pp266–72.

Bowie P & Mountain G, 1993, 'Using Direct Observation to Record the Behaviour of Long-Stay Patients with Dementia', *International Journal of Geriatric Psychiatry* 8, pp857–64.

Brayne C & Calloway P, 1989, 'An Epidemiological Study of Dementia in a Rural Population of Elderly Women', *British Journal of Psychiatry* 155, pp214–19.

Briscoe T, 1990, 'Activity and Stimulation Therapies', Stokes G & Goudie F (eds), *Working with Dementia,* Winslow Press, Bicester.

Brody E, Kleban M, Powell Lawton M & Silverman H, 1971, 'Excess Disabilities of the Mentally Impaired Aged: the Impact of Individualised Treatment', *The Gerontologist* 11, pp124–33.

Brooker DJR, Sturmey P, Gatherer AJH & Sumerbell C, 1993, 'The Behavioural Assessment Scale of Later Life (BASOLL): a Description, Factor Analysis, Scale Development, Validity and Reliability Data For a New Scale for Older Adults', *International Journal of Geriatric Psychiatry* 8, pp747–54.

Brooker DJR, Snape M, Johnson E, Ward D & Payne M, 1997, 'Single Case Evaluation of the Effects of Aromatherapy and Massage on Disturbed Behaviour in Severe Dementia', *British Journal of Clinical Psychology* 36, pp 287–96.

Bryan K & Maxim J, 1994, 'How Not To Give As Good As You Get', *Journal of Dementia Care* 2, pp25–7.

Buckland S, 1997, 'How Well is Well-Being in Dementia?', *PSIGE Newsletter* 60, pp8–10.

Burgener SC, Jirovec M, Murrell L & Barton D, 1992, 'Caregiver and Environmental Variables Related to Difficult Behaviours in Institutionalized Demented Elderly Persons', *Journal of Gerontology* 47, pp242–9.

Burleigh S & Armstrong C, 1997, 'On the Scent of a Useful Therapy', *Journal of Dementia Care* 5, pp21–3.

Burns A, Jacoby R & Levy R, 1990a, 'Psychiatric Phenomena in Alzheimer's Disease I: Disorders of Thought Content', *British Journal of Psychiatry* 157, pp72–6.

Burns A, Jacoby R, & Levy R, 1990b, 'Psychiatric Phenomena in Alzheimer's Disease II: Disorders of Perception', *British Journal of Psychiatry* 157, pp76–81.

Burns A, Jacoby R, & Levy R, 1990c, 'Psychiatric Phenomena in Alzheimer's Disease IV: Disorders of Behaviour', *British Journal of Psychiatry* 157, pp86–94.

Burnside IM, 1980, *Nursing Care of the Aged, 2nd edn,* McGraw-Hill, New York.

Byrne EJ, 1987, 'Reversible Dementia', *International Journal of Geriatric Psychiatry* 2, pp73–81.

Byrne EJ, Lennox G, Low J & Goodwin-Austen RB, 1989, 'Diffuse Lewy Body Disease, Clinical Features in 15 cases', *Journal of Neurology, Neurosurgery and Psychiatry* 5, pp709–17.

Carr EG, 1988, 'Giving Away the Behavioural Approach', *Behavioural Psychotherapy* 16, pp78–84.

Chenoweth B & Spencer B, 1986, 'Dementia: The Experience of Family Caregivers', *The Gerontologist* 26, pp267–72.

Clarke M, Jagger C, Anderson J, Battcock T, Kelly F & Campbell Stern M, 1991, 'The Prevalence of Dementia in a Total Population: a Comparison of Two Screening Instruments', *Age and Ageing* 20, pp396–403.

Cohen-Mansfield J & Werner P, 1997, 'Typology of Disruptive Vocalizations in Older Persons Suffering from Dementia', *International Journal of Geriatric Psychiatry* 12, pp1079–91.

Cohen-Mansfield J, Marx MS & Werner P, 1989, 'Full Moon: Does it Influence Agitated Nursing Home Residents?', *Journal of Clinical Psychology* 45, pp611–14.

Cohen-Mansfield J, Werner P & Marx MS, 1992, 'The Social Environment of the Agitated Nursing Home Resident', *International Journal of Geriatric Psychiatry* 7, pp789–98.

Colerick EJ & George LK, 1986, 'Predictors of Institutionalization Among Caregivers of Patients with Alzheimer's disease', *Journal of the American Geriatric Society* 34, pp493–98.

Colling J, Ouslander J, Hadley BJ, Eish J & Campbell E, 1992, 'The Effects of Patterned Urge-Response Toileting (PURT) on Urinary Incontinence Among Nursing Home Residents', *Journal of the American Geriatrics Society* 40(2), pp 135–41.

Cooney C & Howard R, 1995, 'Abuse of Patients with Dementia by Carers – Out of Sight But Not Out of Mind', *International Journal of Geriatric Psychiatry* 10, pp735–41.

Copeland JRM, Kelleher MJ, Kellett JM *et al,* 1976. 'A Semi-Structured Clinical Interview for the Assessment of Diagnosis and Mental State in the Elderly: The Geriatric Mental State Schedule I. Development and Reliability', *Psychological Medicine* 16, pp89–99.

Coyne A, Reichman W & Berbig L, 1993, 'The Relationship between Dementia and Elder Abuse', *American Journal of Psychiatry* 150, pp643–46.

Crimmens P, 1995, 'Beyond Words: To the Core of Human Need for Contact', *Journal of Dementia Care* 3, pp12–14.

Cummings J, 1985, 'Organic Delusions: Phenomenology, Anatomical Correlations and Review', *British Journal of Psychiatry* 146, pp 184–97.

Cummings J & Benson DF, 1983, *Dementia: A Clinical Approach,* Butterworths, Boston.

Dean R, Briggs K & Lindesay J, 1993, 'The Domus Philosophy: A Prospective Evaluation of Two Residential Units for the Elderly Mentally Ill', *International Journal of Geriatric Psychiatry* 8, pp807–17.

Deutsch LH, Bylsma FW, Rovner BW, Steele CS & Folstein MF, 1991, 'Psychosis and Physical Aggression in Probable Alzheimer's Disease', *American Journal of Psychiatry* 148, pp1159–63.

De Leon MJ, Potegal M & Gurland B, 1984, 'Wandering and Parietal Signs in Senile Dementia of Alzheimer's Disease', *Neuropsychobiology* 11, pp155–7.

Dickinson J, McLain-Kark J & Marshall-Baker A, 1995, 'The Effects of Visual Barriers on Existing Behaviour in a Dementia Care Unit', *The Gerontologist* 35, pp126–30.

Dietch JT, Hewett LJ & Jones S, 1989, 'Adverse Effects of Reality Orientation', *Journal of the American Geriatric Society* 37, pp974–6.

Dodds P, 1994, 'Wandering: A Short Report on Coping Strategies Adopted by Informal Carers', *International Journal of Geriatric Psychiatry* 9, pp751–6.

Dowling Z, Baker R, Wareing LA & Assey J, 1997, 'Lights, Sound and Special Effects?', *Journal of Dementia Care* 5 (1), pp16–18.

Duncan-Jones P & Henderson S, 1978, 'The Use of A Two-Phase Design in a Population Survey', *Social Psychiatry* 13, pp231–7.

Eagles JM, Beattie JAG, Blackwood GW et al, 1987, 'The Mental Health of Elderly Couples – I: The Effects of the Cognitively Impaired Spouse', *British Journal of Psychiatry* 150, pp293–8.

Eastley R & Wilcock GK, 1997, 'Prevalence and Correlates of Aggressive Behaviours Occurring in Patients with Alzheimer's Disease', *International Journal of Geriatric Psychiatry* 12, pp484–7.

Emerson E, 1993, 'Challenging Behaviours and Severe Learning Disabilities: Recent Developments in Behavioural Analysis and Intervention', *Behavioural and Cognitive Psychotherapy* 21, pp171–98.

Enderby P, 1990, 'Promoting Communication in Patients with Dementia', Stokes G & Goudie F (eds), *Working with Dementia,* Winslow Press, Bicester.

Erikson EH, 1963, *Childhood and Society*, 2nd edn, Norton, New York.

Esquirol JED, 1838 (1976), *Des Malades Mentales,* vol 2, Arno, New York.

Fairburn CG & Hope RA, 1988, 'Changes in Behaviour in Dementia: A Neglected Research Area', *British Journal of Psychiatry* 152, pp406–7.

Fallowfield L, 1990, *The Quality of Life: The Missing Measurement in Health Care,* Souvenir Press, London.

Feil N, 1967, 'Group Therapy in a Home for the Aged', *The Gerontologist* 7, pp192–5.

Feil N, 1972, 'A New Approach to Group Therapy', unpublished paper, presented to the Gerontological Society Annual Meeting, San Juan, Puerto Rico.

Feil N, 1992, *Validation: The Feil Method,* Edward Feil Productions, Cleveland.

Fisher JE & Carstensen LL, 1990, 'Behaviour Management of the Dementias', *Clinical Psychology Review* 10, pp611–29.

Folsom JC, 1967, 'Intensive Hospital Therapy of Geriatric Patients', *Current Psychiatric Therapy* 7, pp209–15.

Folsom JC, 1968, 'Reality Orientation Therapy for the Elderly Mental Patient', *Journal of Geriatric Psychiatry* 1, pp291–307.

Folstein ME, Folstein SE & McHugh PR, 1975, 'Mini-Mental State: A Practical Method for Grading the Cognitive State of Patient for Clinician', *Journal of Psychiatry Research* 12, pp189–98.

Fox L, 1995, 'Mapping the Advance of the New Culture in Dementia Care', Kitwood T & Benson S (eds), *The New Culture of Dementia Care,* Hawker Publications, London.

Frank BA, 1995, 'People with Dementia Can Communicate – If We are Able To Hear', Kitwood T & Benson S (eds), *The New Culture of Dementia Care,* Hawker Publications, London.

Freyne A, Kidd N & Lawlor BA, 1998, 'Early Onset Dementia – A Catchment Area Study of Prevalence and Clinical Characteristics', *Irish Journal of Psychological Medicine* 15, pp87–90

Frogatt A, 1994, 'Tuning into Spiritual Needs', *Journal of Dementia Care* 2, pp12–13.

George LK & Gwyther LP, 1986, 'Caregiver Well-being: A Multidimensional Examination of Family Caregivers of Demented Adults', *The Gerontologist* 26, pp253–9.

Ghaziuddin N & McDonald C, 1985, 'A Clinical Study of Adult Copraphagics', *British Journal of Psychiatry* 147, pp312–13.

Gibson F, Marley J & McVicker H, 1995, 'Through the Past to the Person', *Journal of Dementia Care* 3 (6), pp18–19.

Gilhooly MLM, 1984 'The Impact of Caregiving on Caregivers: Factors Associated with the Psychological Well-Being of People Supporting a Dementing Relative in the Community', *British Journal of Medical Psychology* 57, pp35–44.

Gilleard CJ, 1984, *Living with Dementia,* Croom Helm, London.

Gilleard CJ & Watt G, 1982, 'The Impact of Psychogeriatric Day Care on the Primary Supporter of the Elderly Mentally Infirm', Taylor R & Gilmore D (eds), *Current Trends in British Gerontology,* Gower, Aldershot.

Gilleard CJ, Mitchell RG & Riordan J, 1981, 'Ward Orientation Training with Psychogeriatric Patients', *Journal of Advanced Nursing* 6, pp95–8.

Gilleard CJ, Boyd WD & Watt G, 1982, 'Problems in Caring for the Elderly Mentally Infirm at Home', *Archives of Gerontology and Geriatrics* I, pp151–8.

Gilleard CJ, Belford H, Gilleard E, Whittick JE & Gledhill A, 1984, 'Emotional Distress Among the Supporters of the Elderly Mentally Infirm', *British Journal of Psychiatry* 145, pp172–7.

Goldiamond I, 1974, 'Toward a Constructional Approach to Social Problems: Ethical and Constitutional Issues Raised by Applied Behaviour Analysis', *Behaviourism* 2, pp1–84.

Goodall M, 1997, 'Let There Be Light', *The Journal of Dementia Care* 5 (1), pp25–26.

Goodall A, Drage T & Bell G, 1994, *The Bereavement and Loss Training Manual,* Winslow Press, Bicester.

Gormley N, Rizwan MR & Lovestone S, 1998, 'Clinical Predictors of Aggressive Behaviour in Alzheimer's Disease', *International Journal of Geriatric Psychiatry* 13, pp109–15.

Goudie F, 1990, 'Goal Planning: Towards Meeting Individual Needs', Stokes G & Goudie F (eds), *Working with Dementia,* Winslow Press, Bicester.

Goudie F & Stokes G, 1989, 'Understanding Confusion', *Nursing Times* 85 (39), pp35–37.

Goudie F, Bennett R & Steed A, 1990, 'The Maintenance of Independence', Stokes G & Goudie F (eds), *Working with Dementia,* Winslow Press, Bicester.

Grad J & Sainsbury P, 1965, 'An Evaluation of the Effects of Caring for the Aged at Home', *Psychiatric Disorders in the Aged,* WPA Symposium, Geigy, Manchester.

Granacher RP, 1982, 'Agitation in the Elderly. An Often Treatable Manifestation of Acute Brain Syndrome', *Postgraduate Medicine* 72, pp83–96.

Greene JG, Smith R, Gardiner M & Timbury GC, 1982, 'Measuring Behavioural Disturbance of Elderly Demented Patients in the Community and Its Effects on Relatives: A Factor Analytic Study', *Age and Ageing* 11, pp121–6.

Hachinski VC, Lassen NA & Marshall J, 1974, 'Multi-Infarct Dementia: A Cause of Mental Deterioration in the Elderly', *The Lancet* 2, pp207–9.

Haddad PM & Benbow SM, 1993a, 'Sexual Problems Associated with Dementia: Part 1. Problems and their Consequences' *International Journal of Geriatric Psychiatry* 8, pp547–51.

Haddad PM & Benbow SM, 1993b, 'Sexual Problems Associated with Dementia: Part 2. Aetiology, Assessment and Treatment', *International Journal of Geriatric Psychiatry,* 8, pp631–7.

Hamel M, Gold DP, Andres D, Reis M, Dastoor D, Graver H & Bergman H, 1990, 'Prediction and Consequences of Aggressive Behaviour by Community. Based Dementia Patients', *The Gerontologist* 30, pp206–11.

Handysides S, 1993, 'Helping People with Dementia Feel at Home', *British Medical Journal* 306, pp1115–17.

Hanley I, McGuire RJ & Boyd WD, 1981, 'Reality Orientation and Dementia: A Controlled Trial of Two Approaches', *British Journal of Psychiatry* 138, pp10–14.

Harding J, 1995, *Design for Dementia, Arts for Health,* Manchester Metropolitan University, Manchester.

Harding J & Jolley D, 1994, 'Design for Dementia', *HD,* November, pp21–3.

Hebb DO, 1955, Drives and the CNS (Conceptual Nervous System)', *Psychology Review* 62, pp243–54.

Henderson AS, 1983, 'The Coming Epidemic of Dementia', *Australian and New Zealand Journal of Psychiatry* 17, pp117–27.

Henderson AS, 1986, 'The Epidemiology of Alzheimer's Disease', *British Medical Bulletin* 42, pp3–10.

Henderson AS, 1987, 'Alzheimer's Disease: Epidemiology', Pitt B (ed), *Dementia,* Churchill Livingstone, Edinburgh.

Henderson AS & Jorm AF, 1986, *The Problem of Dementia in Australia,* Australian Government Publishing Service, Canberra.

Hewawasum L, 1996, 'Floor Patterns Limit Wandering of People with Alzheimer's', *Nursing Times* 92 (23), pp41–4.

Hodge J, 1984, 'Towards a Behavioural Analysis of Dementia', Hanley I & Hodge J (eds), *Psychological Approaches to the Care of the Elderly,* Croom Helm, London.

Hofman A, Rocca WA, Brayne C *et al,* 1991, 'The Prevalence of Dementia in Europe: A Collaborative Study of 1980–1990 Findings', *International Journal of Epidemiology* 20 (3), pp736–48.

Holden UP, 1987, 'The Value of Reality Orientation in 1987', *Clinical Rehabilitation* 1, pp235–8.

Holden UP, 1990a, 'Dementia: Some Common Misunderstandings', Stokes G & Goudie F (eds), *Working with Dementia,* Winslow Press, Bicester.

Holden UP, 1990b, 'Neuropsychological Deficits. Rehabilitation and Retraining', Stokes G & Goudie F (eds), *Working with Dementia,* Winslow Press, Bicester.

Holden UP, 1990c, 'Reality Orientation in the 1990s', Stokes G & Goudie F (eds), *Working with Dementia,* Winslow Press, Bicester.

Holden UP, 1995, *Ageing, Neuropsychology and the 'New' Dementias,* Chapman & Hall, London.

Holden UP & Woods RT, 1982, *Reality Orientation: Psychological Approaches to the Confused Elderly,* Churchill Livingstone, Edinburgh.

Hook M, 1998, *Gentle Exercises and Movement for Frail People,* Winslow Press, Bicester.

Hooper J, 1994, 'Shaking a Stick at Fear', *Journal of Dementia Care,* 2 (2), pp22–3.

Hope RA & Fairburn CG, 1990, 'The Nature of Wandering in Dementia: A Community Based Study', *International Journal of Geriatric Psychiatry* 5, pp239–45.

Hope RA & Fairburn CG, 1992, 'The Present Behavioural Examination (PBE): The Development of an Interview to Measure Current Behavioural Abnormalities', *Psychological Medicine* 22, pp223–30.

Hope RA & Patel V, 1993, 'Assessment of Behavioural Phenomena in Dementia', Burns A (ed), *Ageing and Dementia: A Methodological Approach,* Edward Arnold, London.

Hope RA, Fairburn CG & Goodwin GM, 1989, 'Increased Eating in Dementia', *International Journal of Eating Disorders* 8, pp111–15.

Hope RA, Tilling KM, Gedling K, Keene JM, Cooper SD & Fairburn CG, 1994, 'The Structure of Wandering in Dementia', *International Journal of Geriatric Psychiatry* 9, pp149–55.

Hope RA, Keane J, Fairburn C, McShane R & Jacoby R, 1997, 'Behaviour Changes in Dementia II: Are There Behavioural Syndromes?', *International Journal of Geriatric Psychiatry* 5, pp239–45.

Horowitz A, 1997, 'The Relationship Between Vision Impairment and the Assessment of Disruptive Behaviours Among Nursing Home Residents', *The Gerontologist* 37, pp620–8.

Huppert FA & Tym E, 1986, 'Clinical and Neuropsychological Assessment of Dementia', *British Medical Bulletin* 42 (1), pp11–18.

Hussian RA, 1981, *Geriatric Psychology: A Behavioural Perspective,* Van Nostrand Reinhold, New York.

Hussian RA, 1982, 'Stimulus Control in the Modification of Problematic Behaviour in Elderly Institutionalised Patients', *International Journal of Behavioural Geriatrics* 1, pp33–46.

Hussian RA, 1988, 'Modification of Behaviours in Dementia via Stimulus Manipulation', *Clinical Gerontologist* 8, pp37–43.

Hussian RA & Brown DC, 1987, 'Use of Two Dimensional Grid Pattern to Limit Hazardous Ambulation in Demented Patients', *Journal of Gerontology* 43, pp558–60.

Ikeda M, Mori E, Hirono N *et al,* 1998, 'Amnestic People with Alzheimer's Disease Who Remembered the Kobe Earthquake', *British Journal of Psychiatry* 172, pp425–8.

Inness A, 1998, 'Behind Labels: What Makes Behaviour Difficult?', *Journal of Dementia Care* 6 (5), pp22–5.

Irving M, 1996, 'Handles on Reality', *Sunday Telegraph,* July.

Jagger C & Lindesay J, 1993, 'The Epidemiology of Senile Dementia', Burns A (ed), *Ageing and Dementia: A Methodological Approach,* Edward Arnold, London.

Jensen CF, 1989, 'Hypersexual Agitation in Alzheimer's Disease', *Journal of the American Geriatrics Society* 37, p917.

Jerrom B, Mian I & Rukanyake NG, 1993, 'Stress on Relative Caregivers of Dementia Sufferers and Predictors of the Breakdown of Community Care', *International Journal of Geriatric Psychiatry* 8, pp331–7.

Jorm AF, 1987, *Understanding Senile Dementia,* Croom Helm, London.

Jorm AF, 1990, *The Epidemiology of Alzheimer's Disease and Related Disorders,* Chapman & Hall, London.

Jorm AF & Korten AE, 1988, 'A Method of Calculating Increases in the Number of Dementia Sufferers', *Australian and New Zealand Journal of Psychiatry* 22, pp183–9.

Jorm AF, Korten AE & Henderson AS, 1987, 'The Prevalence of Dementia: A Quantitative Integration of the Literature', *Acta Psychiatrica Scandinavica* 76, pp465–79.

Judd S, 1998, 'Building for Dementia: A Matter of Design', Judd S, Marshall M & Phippen P (eds), *Design for Dementia,* Hawker Publications, London.

Kay DWK & Bergmann K, 1980, 'Epidemiology of Mental Disorders Among the Aged in the Community', Birren JE & Sloane RB (eds), *Handbook of Mental Health and Ageing,* Prentice Hall, Englewood Cliffs.

Keady J, Nolan M & Gilliard J, 1995, 'Listen to the Voices of Experience', *Journal of Dementia Care* 3 (3), pp15–17.

Keen J, 1989, 'Interiors: Architecture in the Lives of People with Dementia', *International Journal of Geriatric Psychiatry* 4, pp255–72.

Killick J, 1994, 'Giving Shape to Shadows', *Elderly Care* 6, p10.

Kingston P & Reay A, 1996, 'Elder Abuse and Neglect', Woods RT (ed), *Handbook of the Clinical Psychology of Ageing,* John Wiley, Chichester.

Kinney JM & Paris Stephens MA, 1989, 'Caregiving Hassles Scale: Assessing the Severity Hassles of Caring for a Family Member with Dementia', *The Gerontologist* 29, pp328–32.

Kitwood T, 1989, 'Brain, Mind and Dementia: With Particular Reference to Alzheimer's Disease', *Ageing and Society* 9, pp1–15.

Kitwood T, 1990, 'The Dialectics of Dementia: With Particular Reference to Alzheimer's Disease', *Ageing and Society* 10, pp177–96.

Kitwood T, 1993, 'Person and Process in Dementia', *International Journal of Geriatric Psychiatry* 9, pp 541–5.

Kitwood T, 1994, 'Lowering Our Defences by Playing the Part', *Journal of Dementia Care* 2, pp12–14.

Kitwood T, 1995, 'Cultures of Care: Tradition and Change', Kitwood T & Benson S (eds), *The New Culture of Dementia Care,* Hawker Publications, London.

Kitwood T, 1996, 'A Dialectical Framework for Dementia', Woods RT (ed), *Handbook of the Clinical Psychology of Ageing,* John Wiley, Chichester.

Kitwood R, 1997, *Dementia Reconsidered,* Open University Press, London.

Kitwood T & Bredin K, 1992, *Person to Person,* Gale Centre Publications, Loughton.

Kitwood T, Buckland S & Petre T, 1995, *Brighter Futures,* Anchor Housing Association, Kidlington.

de Klerk-Rubin V, 1994, 'Misunderstandings About Validation', *Journal of Dementia Care* 2 (2), pp14–16.

Koch T & Webb C, 1996, ' The Biomedical Construction of Ageing: Implications for Nursing Care of Older People', *Journal of Advanced Nursing* 23, pp954–9.

Kral VA, 1962, 'Senescent Forgetfulness: Benign and Malignant', *Canadian Medical Association Journal* 86, pp257–60.

Kral VA, 1978, 'Benign Senescent Forgetfulness', *Ageing* 7, pp47–51.

Lam DH & Woods RT, 1986 'Ward Orientation Training in Dementia: A Single Case Study', *International Journal of Geriatric Psychiatry* 1, pp145–7.

La Vigna GW & Donnellan AM, 1986, *Alternatives to Punishment: Solving Behaviour Problems with Non-Aversive Strategies,* Irvington, New York.

Lawton MP & Simon B, 1968, 'The Ecology of Social Relationships in Housing for the Elderly', *Gerontologist* 8, pp108–15.

Lazarus RS & Delongis A, 1983, 'Psychological Stress and Coping in Ageing', *American Psychologist* 38, pp245–54.

Leng N, 1982, 'Behavioural Treatment of the Elderly', *Age and Ageing* 11, pp235–43.

Lindesay J & Murphy E, 1989, 'Dementia, Depression and Subsequent Institututionalization – The Effect of Home Support', *International Journal of Geriatric Psychiatry* 4, pp3–9.

Lindesay J, Briggs K, Lawes M, MacDonald A & Herzberg J, 1991, 'The Domus Philosophy: A Comparative Evaluation of a New Approach to Residential Care for the Demented Elderly', *International Journal of Geriatric Psychiatry* 6, pp727–36.

Lindsley OR, 1964, 'Geriatric Behavioural Prosthetics', Kastenbaum R (ed), *New Thoughts on Old Age,* Springer, New York.

Lion JR, Snyder W & Merrill GL, 1981, 'Under-reporting of Assaults on Staff in a State Hospital', *Hospital and Community Psychiatry* 32, pp497–8.

Lishman WA, 1987, *Organic Psychiatry*, 2nd edn, Blackwell Scientific, Oxford.

Lovell BB, Ancoli-Israel S & Gevirtz, 1995, 'Effect of Bright Light Treatment on Agitated Behaviour in Institutuionalized Elderly Subjects', *Psychiatry Research* 57, pp7–12.

MacDonald C & Teven T, 1997, *Who's In Control? – A Pilot Study Examining And Questioning The Use Of Anti-Psychotic Drugs In People With Dementia Who Exhibit Challenging Behaviours,* Dementia Services Development Centre, Stirling.

Mace NL & Rabins PV, 1992, *The 36–Hour Day,* Age Concern/Hodder & Stoughton, London.

Machin E, 1980, 'A Survey of the Behaviour of the Elderly and their Supporters at Home', unpublished MSc thesis, University of Birmingham.

Magai C, Cohen CI, Culver C, Gomberg D & Malatesta C, 1997, 'Relation Between PreMorbid Personality and Patterns of Emotion Expression in Mid-to-Late-Stage Dementia', *International Journal of Geriatric Psychiatry* 12, pp1092–9.

Marshall M, 1995, 'Technology is the Shape of the Future', *Journal of Dementia Care* 3 (3), pp12–14.

Marshall M, 1998, 'Therapeutic Buildings for People with Dementia', Judd S, Marshall M & Phippen P (eds), *Design For Dementia,* Hawker Publications, London.

Mayer R & Darby SJ, 1991, 'Does a Mirror Deter Wandering in Demented Older People?', *International Journal of Geriatric Psychiatry* 6, pp607–9.

McKeith I, Fairbairn A, Perry R, Thompson P & Perry E, 1992, 'Neuroleptic Sensitivity in Patients with Senile Dementia of Lewy Body Type', *British Medical Journal* 305, pp673–8.

McKhann G, Drachman D, Folstein M et al, 1984, 'Clinical Diagnosis of Alzheimer's Disease: Report of the NINCDS – ADRDA Work Group, Department of Health and Human Services Task Force on Alzheimer's Disease', *Neurology* 34, pp939–44.

McShane R, 1994, 'Walking or Wandering?', *Journal of Dementia Care* 2 (5), pp24–5.

McShane R, Hope T & Wilkinson J, 1994, 'Tracking Patients Who Wander: Ethics and Technology', *The Lancet* 343, p1274.

Merriam A, Aronson N, Gaston P, Wey S & Katz I, 1988, 'The Psychiatric Symptoms of Alzheimer's Disease', *Journal of the American Geriatric Society* 36, pp7–12.

Merry T, 1995, *Invitation to Person Centred Psychology,* Whurr Publishers, London.

Meyer J, Schalock R & Genaidy H, 1991, 'Aggression in Psychiatric Hospitalized Geriatric Patients', *International Journal of Geriatric Psychiatry* 6, pp589–92.

Miesen BML, 1993, 'Alzheimer's Disease. The Phenomenon of Parent Fixation and Bowlby's Attachment Theory', *International Journal of Geriatric Psychiatry* 8, pp147–53.

Miller BL, Darby A, Benson DF, Cummings JL & Miller MH, 1997, 'Aggressive, Socially Disruptive and Antisocial Behaviour Associated with Fronto-Temporal Dementia', *British Journal of Psychiatry* 170, pp150–5.

Miller E, 1977, *Abnormal Ageing,* John Wiley, London.

Miller E, 1987, 'Reality Orientation with Psychogeriatric Patients: The Limitations', *Clinical Rehabilitation* 1, pp231–3.

Moffitt L, 1996, 'Helping to Re-create a Personal Sacred Space', *Journal of Dementia Care* 4 (3), pp19–21.

Moniz-Cook E, 1998, 'Psychosocial Approaches to 'Challenging Behaviour' in Care Homes', *Journal of Dementia Care* 6 (5), pp33–8.

Moniz-Cook E & Gill, 1996, 'Howling Dogs and Whistling Women', *Journal of Dementia Care* 4 (3), pp16–18.

Moniz-Cook E, Stokes G & Agar S, 1999, 'Difficult Behaviour and Dementia in Nursing Homes: Five Cases of Psychosocial Intervention', *International Journal of Clinical Psychology and Psychotherapy.*

Morgan K & Gledhill K, 1991, *Managing Sleep and Insomnia in the Older Person,* Winslow Press, Bicester (OP).

Morley JE & Silver AJ, 1988, 'Anorexia in the Elderly', *Neurobiology and Ageing* 9, pp9–16.

Morris E, 1995, 'This Living Hand', *The New Yorker,* 16 January, pp66–9.

Morris CH, Hope RA & Fairburn CG, 1989, 'Eating Habits in Dementia: A Descriptive Study, *British Journal of Psychiatry* 154, pp801–6.

Morris LW, Morris RG & Britton PG, 1988, 'The Relationship Between Marital Intimacy, Perceived Strain and Depression in Spouse Carers of Dementia Sufferers', *British Journal of Medical Psychology* 61, pp231–6.

Morris RG & Morris LW, 1993, 'Psychological Aspects of Caring for People with Dementia: Conceptual and Methodological Issues', Burns A (ed), *Ageing and Dementia: A Methodological Approach,* Edward Arnold, London.

243

Morris RG, Woods RT, Davies KS et al, 1992, 'The Use of Coping Strategy Focused Support Group for Carers of Dementia Sufferers', *Counselling Psychology Quarterly* 5 (4), pp 337–48.

Mortimer JA, 1983, 'Alzheimer's Disease and Senile Dementia: Prevalence and Incidence', Reisberg B (ed), *Alzheimer's Disease,* The Free Press, New York.

Mortimer JA, Schuman LM & French LR, 1981, 'Epidemiology of Dementing Illness', Mortimer JA & Schuman LM (eds), *The Epidemiology of Dementia,* Oxford University Press, New York.

Morton I, 1997, 'Beyond Validation', Norman IJ & Redfern SJ (eds), *Mental Healthcare for Elderly People,* Churchill Livingstone, Edinburgh.

Morton I, 2000, *Person-Centred Approaches to Dementia Care,* Winslow Press, Bicester.

Morton I & Bleathman C, 1988, 'Reality Orientation: Does It Matter Whether It's Tuesday or Friday?', *Nursing Times* 84 (6), pp25–7.

Morton I & Bleathman C, 1991, 'The Effectiveness of Validation Therapy in Dementia – a Pilot Study', *International Journal of Geriatric Psychiatry* 6, pp327–30.

Morton I & Bleathman C, 1995, 'The Roots and Growth of Person-Centred Care', *Journal of Dementia Care* 3, pp22–5.

Murphy E, 1986, *Dementia and Mental Illness in the Old,* Papermac, London.

Murphy E, 1991, *After The Asylums,* Faber & Faber, London.

Näsman B, Bucht G, Eriksson S & Sandman PO, 1993, 'Behavioural Symptoms in the Institutionalised Elderly – Relationship to Dementia', *International Journal of Geriatric Psychiatry* 8, pp843–9.

Netten A, 1989, 'The Effect of Design of Residential Homes in Creating Dependency Among Confused Elderly Residents', *International Journal of Geriatric Psychiatry* 4, pp143–53.

O'Connor M, 1987, 'Disturbed Behaviour in Dementia: Psychiatric or Medical Problem', *Medical Journal of Australia* 147, pp 481–5.

Ogg J & Bennett GCJ, 1992, 'Elder Abuse in Britain', *British Medical Journal* 305, pp998–9.

Pagel MD, Becker J & Cappel DB, 1985, 'Loss of Control, Self-Blame and Depression, An Investigation of Spouse Caregivers of Alzheimer's Disease Patients', *Journal of Abnormal Psychology* 94, pp169–82.

Palmer AM, Stratmann GC, Proctor AW & Bowen DM, 1988, 'Possible Neurotransmitter Basis of Behavioural Changes in Alzheimer's Disease', *Annals of Neurology* 23, pp616–20.

Pastalan L, 1984, 'Architectural Research and Life-Space Changes', Snyder J (ed), *Architectural Research,* Van Nostrand Reinhold, New York.

Patel V & Hope RA, 1992a, 'Aggressive Behaviour in a Hospitalised Psychogeriatric Population', *Acta Psychiatrica Scandinavica* 85, pp131–5.

Patel V & Hope RA, 1992b, 'A Rating Scale for Aggressive Behaviour in the Elderly (the RAGE)', *Psychological Medicine* 22, pp211–21.

Patel V & Hope RA, 1993, 'Aggressive behaviour in Elderly People with Dementia: A Review', *International Journal of Geriatric Psychiatry* 8, pp457–72.

Patterson, CH, 1984, 'Empathy, Warmth and Genuineness in Psychotherapy: A review of Reviews', *Psychotherapy* 21, pp431–8.

Patterson RL, Dupree LW, Eberly DA *et al*, 1982, *Overcoming Deficits of Ageing: A Behavioural Approach,* Plenum Press, New York.

Pattie A, 1988, 'Measuring Levels of Disability – The Clifton Assessment Procedures for the Elderly', Wattis JP & Hindmarch I (eds), *Psychological Assessment of the Elderly,* Churchill Livingstone, Edinburgh.

Pattie A & Gilleard CJ, 1979, *Manual of the Clifton Assessment Procedures for the Elderly* (cape), Hodder & Stoughton, Sevenoaks.

Pennington R, 1996, 'Blowing the Whistle on Bad Design', *Journal of Dementia Care* 3, pp24–6.

Perrin T, 1995, 'A New Pattern of Life: Re-assessing the Role of Occupation and Activities', Kitwood T & Benson S (eds), *The New Culture of Dementia Care,* Hawker Publications, London.

Perrin T, 1996, *Problem Behaviour and the Care of Elderly People,* Winslow Press, Bicester.

Petrie WM, Lawson EC & Hollender, MH, 1982, 'Violence in Geriatric Patients', *Journal of the American Medical Association* 248, pp443–4.

Pick A, 1904, 'Zur Symptomatologie der Linksseitigen Schlafenlappenatrophie', *Monatschrift für Psychiatrie und Neurologie* 16, pp378–88.

Pillemer KA & Moore DW, 1989, 'Abuse of Patients in Nursing Homes: Findings From a Staff Survey', *The Gerontologist* 29, pp314–20.

Pitt B, 1987, 'Delirium and Dementia', Pitt B (ed), *Dementia,* Churchill Livingstone, Edinburgh.

Poulshock SW & Deimling GT, 1984, 'Families Caring for Elders in Residence: Issues in the Measurement of Burden', *Journal of Gerontology* 39, pp230–9.

Prouty G, 1994, *Theoretical Evolutions in Person-Centred Experiential Therapy: Applications to Schizophrenic and Retarded Psychoses,* Praeger, Westport.

Pruchno RA & Resch NL, 1989, 'Aberrant behaviours and Alzheimer's Disease: Mental Health Effects on Spouse Caregivers' *Journal of Gerontology* 44, pp177–82.

Rabins PV, Mace HL & Lucas MJ, 1982, 'The Impact of Dementia on the Family', *Journal of the American Medical Association* 248, pp333–5.

Reisberg B, Borenstein J, Salob S, Ferris S, Franssen E & Georgotas A, 1987, 'Behavioural Symptoms in Alzheimer's Disease: Phenomenology and treatment', *Journal of Clinical Psychiatry* 48, Suppl. 5 (May), pp9–15.

Rogers CR, 1951, *Client-Centred Therapy: Its Current Practice, Implications and Theory,* Houghton Mifflin, Boston.

Rogers CR, 1957, 'The Necessary and Sufficient Conditions of Therapeutic Personality Change', *Journal of Consulting Psychology* 21, pp95–103.

Rogers CR, 1980, *A Way of Being,* Houghton Mifflin, Boston.

Rogers CR, 1986, 'Reflection of Feelings', *Person-Centred Review* I, pp125–40.

Rorsman B, Hagnell O & Lanke J, 1986, 'Prevalence and Incidence of Senile and Multi- Infarct Dementia in the Lundby Study: A Comparison Between Time Periods 1947–1957 and 1957–1972', *Neuropsychobiology* 15, pp122–9.

Roth M, Huppert FA, Tym E & Mountjoy CQ, 1988, *The Cambridge Mental Disorders of the Elderly Examination,* Cambridge University Press, Cambridge.

Royal College of Physicians, 1981, 'Organic Mental Impairment in the Elderly', *Journal of the Royal College of Physicians* 15, pp141–7.

Rubin E, Drevets W & Burke A, 1988, 'The Nature of Psychotic Symptoms in Senile Dementia of the Alzheimer Type', *Journal of Geriatric Psychiatry and Neurology* I, pp16–20.

Ryden MB, 1988, 'Aggressive Behaviour in Persons with Dementia who Live in the Community', *Alzheimer's Disease and Associated Disorder* 2, pp342–5.

Samson DM & McDonnell AA, 1990, 'Functional Analysis and Challenging Behaviours', *Behavioural Psychotherapy* 18, pp259–72.

Sandford JRA, 1975, 'Tolerance of Debility in Elderly Dependants by Supporters at Home: Its Significance for Hospital Practice', *British Medical Journal* 3, pp471–5.

Satlin A, Teicher MH, Leiberman HR *et al,* 1991, 'Circadian Locomotor Activity Rythms in Alzheimer's Disease, *Neuropsychopharmacology* 5, pp22–5.

Sayer RJ, 1994, 'The Management of Wandering in Nursing and Residential Homes: Is There a Role for Occupational Therapy?', *unpublished report,* School of Health and Social Sciences, Coventry University.

Schaffer HR, 1971, *The Growth of Sociability*, Penguin Books, Harmondsworth.

Schneider LS & Sabin PB, 1994, 'Treatments for Psychiatric Symptoms and Behavioural Disturbances in Dementia', Burns A & Levy R (eds), *Dementia,* Chapman & Hall Medical, London.

Seth RV, 1994, 'Review: Weight Loss in Alzheimer's Disease', *International Journal of Geriatric Psychiatry* 9, pp605–10.

Shah AK, 1991, 'Low Levels of Violence on a Psychogeriatric Ward', *Geriatric Medicine* 21, p27.

Shah AK, 1992, 'Violence and Psychogeriatric Inpatients', *International Journal of Geriatric Psychiatry* 7, pp39–44.

Sheldon F, 1982, 'Supporting the Supporters: Working with the Relatives of Patients with Dementia', *Age and Ageing* 11, pp184–8.

Silver JM & Yudofsky SC, 1987, 'Documentation of Aggression in the Assessment of the Violent Patient', *Psychiatric Annals* 17, pp375–84.

Sixsmith A, Stillwell J & Copeland J, 1993, 'Rementia: Challenging The Limits of Dementia Care', *International Journal of Geriatric Psychiatry* 8, pp993–1000.

Smith J, 1994, 'Reading Around ... Risk and Restraint', *Journal of Dementia Care* 2 (1), pp18–19.

Snyder LH, Rupprecht P, Pyrek J, Brekhus S & Moss T, 1978 'Wandering', *The Gerontologist* 18, pp272–80.

Sourander P & Sjogren H, 1970, 'The Concept of Alzheimer's Disease and Its Clinical Implications', Wolstenholme G & O'Connor M (eds), *Alzheimer's Disease and Related Conditions,* Churchill, London.

Spivack M, 1967, 'Sensory Distortion in Tunnels and Corridors', *Hospital and Community Psychiatry* 18, January.

Steele C, Rouner B, Chase GA & Folstein M, 1990, 'Psychiatric Symptoms and Nursing Home Placement of Patients with Alzheimer's Disease, *American Journal of Psychiatry* 147, pp1049–51.

Stokes G, 1986a, *'Common Problems with the Elderly Confused: Wandering,* Winslow Press, Bicester.

Stokes G, 1986b, *Common Problems with the Elderly Confused: Screaming and Shouting,* Winslow Press, Bicester.

Stokes G, 1987a, *Common Problems with the Elderly Confused: Incontinence and Inappropriate Urinating,* Winslow Press, Bicester.

Stokes G, 1987b, *Common Problems with the Elderly Confused: Aggression,* Winslow Press, Bicester.

Stokes G, 1990a, 'Behavioural Analysis', Stokes G & Goudie F (eds), *Working with Dementia,* Winslow Press, Bicester.

Stokes G, 1990b, 'The Environmental Context', Stokes G & Goudie F (eds), *Working with Dementia,* Winslow Press, Bicester.

Stokes G, 1990c, 'The Management of Toileting Difficulties', Stokes G & Goudie F (eds), *Working with Dementia,* Winslow Press, Bicester.

Stokes G, 1990d, 'Controlling Disruptive & Demanding Behaviours', Stokes G & Goudie F (eds), *Working with Dementia,* Winslow Press, Bicester.

Stokes G, 1992, *On Being Old,* Falmer Press, London.

Stokes G, 1995a, 'Incontinent or Not? Don't Label: Describe and Assess', *Journal of Dementia Care* 3 (1), pp20–1.

Stokes G, 1995b, 'Incontinent or Not? Person First, Dementia Second', *Journal of Dementia Care* 3 (2), pp20–1.

Stokes G, 1995c, 'Incontinent or Not? Multi-Modal Therapy', *Journal of Dementia Care* 3 (3), pp17–19.

Stokes G, 1996, 'Driven by Fear to Defend His Secure World', *Journal of Dementia Care* 4 (3), pp14–16.

Stokes G, 1997, 'Reacting to a Real Threat', *Journal of Dementia Care* 5 (1), pp14–15.

Stokes G & Allen B, 1990, 'Seeking an Explanation', Stokes G & Goudie F (eds), *Working with Dementia,* Winslow Press, Bicester.

Stokes G & Goudie F, 1990, 'Confused Elderly People', Stokes G & Goudie F (eds), *Working with Dementia,* Winslow Press, Bicester.

Struble LM & Sivertsen L, 1987, 'Agitation Behaviours in Confused Elderly Patients', *Journal of Gerontological Nursing* 13, pp40–44.

Sunderland T & Silver MA, 1988, 'Neuroleptics in the Treatment of Dementia', *International Journal of Geriatric Psychiatry* 3, pp79–88.

Swaab DF, Fliers E & Partiman TS, 1985, 'The Suprachiasmatic Nucleus of Human Brain in Relation to Sex, Age and Senile Dementia', *Brain Research* 342, pp 37–44

Swearer JM, Drachman DA, O'Donnell B & Mitchell AL, 1988, 'Troublesome and Disruptive behaviours in Dementia – Relationships to Diagnosis and Disease Severity', *Journal of the American Geriatric Society* 36, pp784–90.

Taft LB & Barkin RL, 1990, 'Drug Abuse? Use and Misuse of Psychotropic Drugs in Alzheimer's Disease', *Journal of Gerontological Nursing* 16, pp4–10.

Taulbee LR & Folsom JC, 1966, 'Reality Orientation for Geriatric Patients', *Hospital and Community Psychiatry* 17, pp133–35

Terry RD, 1992, 'The Pathogenesis of Alzheimer's Disease: What Causes Dementia?', Christen Y & Churchland P (eds), *Neurophilosophy and Alzheimer's Disease,* Springer Verlag, Berlin.

Thomas DR, 1988, 'Assessment and Management of Agitation in the Elderly', *Geriatrics* 43, pp45–53.

Tobiansky R, 1995, 'Understanding Dementia', *Journal of Dementia Care* 3 (2), pp27–8.

Townsend P, 1962, *The Last Refuge,* Routledge & Kegan Paul, London.

Trinkle DB, Burns A & Levy R, 1992, 'Brief Report: Abnormal Eating Behaviour in Dementia – A Descriptive Study', *International Journal of Geriatric Psychiatry* 7, pp799–803.

U' Ren R, 1987 'Introduction', Pitt B (ed), *Dementia,* Churchill Livingstone, Edinburgh.

Van Werde D & Morton I, 2000, 'The Relevance of Prouty's Pre-Therapy to Dementia Care', Morton I (ed), *Person-Centred Approaches to Dementia Care,* Winslow Press, Bicester.

Wade JPH & Hachinski VC, 1987, 'Multi-Infarct Dementia', Pitt B (ed), *Dementia,* Churchill Livingstone, Edinburgh.

Ware CJG, Fairburn CG & Hope RA, 1990, 'A Community-Based Study of Aggressive Behaviour in Dementia', *International Journal of Geriatric Psychiatry* 5, pp337–42.

Wattis J, 1990, 'Medication in the Management of Dementia', Stokes G & Goudie F (eds), *Working with Dementia,* Winslow Press, Bicester.

Welsh SW, Corrigan FM & Scott M, 1996 'Language Impairment and Aggression in Alzheimer's Disease', *International Journal of Geriatric Psychiatry* 11, pp257–61.

West BJM & Brockman SJ, 1994, 'The Calming Power of Aromatherapy', *Journal of Dementia Care* 2 (2), pp20–1.

Wetzler MA & Feil N, 1978, *Manual for Implementing the Feil Method,* Edward Feil Productions, Cleveland.

Whalley LJ, Carothers AD, Collyer S, De May R & Frackiewicz A, 1982, 'Familial Factors in Alzheimer's Disease', *British Journal of Psychiatry* 140, pp249–56.

Wolfe N & Herzberg J, 1996, 'Letter to the Editor: Can Aromatherapy Oils Promote Sleep in Severely Demented Patients?' *International Journal of Geriatric Psychiatry* 11, pp926–27.

Woods RT, 1983, 'Specificity of Learning in Reality Orientation Sessions: A Single-Case Study', *Behaviour Research and Therapy* 21, pp173–5.

Woods RT, 1992, 'What Can Be Learned From Studies on Reality Orientation?', Jones GMM & Miesen BM (eds), *Care-Giving in Dementia,* Routledge, London.

Woods RT, 1994, 'Reality Orientation', *Journal of Dementia Care* 2 (2), pp24–5.

Woods RT, 1995, 'The Beginnings of a New Culture in Care', Kitwood T & Benson S (eds) *The New Culture of Dementia Care,* Hawker Publications, London.

Woods RT, 1996, 'Institutional Care', Woods RT (ed) *Handbook of the Clinical Psychology of Ageing,* John Wiley, Chichester.

World Health Organisation, 1982. *World Health Statistics Quarterly* 35 (3&4), WHO, Geneva.

World Health Organisation, 1990, *International Classification of Disease: Mental and Behaviour Disorders, Diagnosis Criteria for Research,* WHO, Geneva.

Yudofsky SC, Silver JM & Hales, RE, 1990, 'Pharmalogic Management of Aggression in the Elderly', *Journal of Clinical Psychiatry* 51, pp22–8.

Zarit SH & Edwards AB, 1996, 'Family Caregiving: Research and Clinical Intervention', Woods RT (ed), *Handbook of the Clinical Psychology of Ageing,* John Wiley, Chichester.

Zarit SH, Todd PA & Zarit JM, 1986, 'Subjective Burden of Husbands and Wives as Caregivers: A Long Titudinal Study', *The Gerontologist* 26, pp260–6.

Index

INDEX